Praise for *125 Best Gluten-Free Recipes*

"Donna and Heather use healthy grains such as whole bean, flaxseed, amaranth, quinoa, rice bran and a variety of seeds and nuts in many of their recipes. They have made their recipes more nutritious by limiting the salt, sugar and fat, while using fresh fruits, vegetables and juices. Make sure you add this book to your collection of gluten-free resources!"

— Shelley Case, B.Sc, RD, consulting dietitian and author of *Gluten-Free Diet: A Comprehensive Resource Guide*

"With this gluten-free cookbook and a little patience and practice, anyone can master the art of cooking gluten-free."

— Mavis Malloy, RDN, dietitian, member of the Professional Advisory Board, Canadian Celiac Association

"We are so excited about the research you have done for us on gluten-free starches and flours. The information on the newer gluten-free flours along with your recipes will be an invaluable tool for parents of celiacs and our dietitians."

— Rochelle Yeo, RD, and Rhonda Karas-Chartrand, RD, Stollery Children's Hospital, Edmonton, Alberta

"I made the Chocolate Fudge Cake (on front cover) for my daughter-in-law's birthday (we are both celiacs) and it was by far the BEST gluten-free cake either of us has ever eaten. Six others who are not celiacs also ate the cake and loved it."

— Juanita A. Ohanian, Celiac Sprue Support Group, Rockville, Maryland

"A great find — so informative, some excellent tips, good variety. Seems Donna and Heather have done their homework on gluten-free cooking. I was really impressed with this book."

— Janet, Maine

"Thanks a million times over for your wonderful cookbook. Thanks to your cookbook, we are eating foods that are like normal foods again. I have tried other gluten-free cookbooks and yours is the best by far!

— Kevin Johnston, California

"This book is chock full of fantastic recipes! People without gluten intolerance rave about the food I have prepared from this book. I highly recommend *125 Best Gluten-Free Recipes*. It has been a lifesaver to me and my family."

— Kristeena Newberg, Superior, Wisconsin

"I attended the chapter meeting and was delighted to hear Donna and Heather speak. Their talk encouraged me immensely and I tried the pie pastry — SUCCESS! I really appreciate the work and testing they put into every recipe in the book, and I no longer feel hesitant about trying them. Thank you so much."

— Sheila E. Green, member, London Chapter, Canadian Celiac Association

"Donna and Heather have elevated gluten-free cooking from relatively boring to delicious, easy-to-prepare recipes, made from easily obtainable ingredients. The book is well laid out, with good sensible information. All the recipes we've tried have been successful and tasty. The glossaries provide useful tips and important information. Their common-sense approach truly helps demystify some of the poorly understood aspects of this disease."

— Henk Rietveld, Huntsville, Ontario

"I am totally impressed with this cookbook. I have adapted recipes and cooked for my celiac husband for over 10 years, and I thought I knew a lot about good gluten-free baking. However, this book has given me a ton of good ideas (and recipes that work) and has rekindled my interest in baking. Another plus is that the recipes are good enough for me (a non-celiac) too! There is a wealth of information about alternative flours."

— Elaine Sorensen, Winfield, British Columbia

"Donna and Heather have a real winner on their hands. They have taken the specialized cooking and baking required for a gluten-free diet and rethought it from starter to dessert. The recipes are innovative, and every one I've tried is delicious. The glossaries, as well as the helpful hints on each recipe, make this a valuable resource book for anyone struggling with gluten-free cooking. The bread recipes include detailed instructions for both machine and mixer, so everyone can accomplish fabulous results. My cookbook library wouldn't be complete without it."

— Sue Jennett, Kingston, Ontario

the Best
Gluten-Free
Family Cookbook

Donna Washburn & Heather Butt

Robert
ROSE

Here's to well-seasoned friendships

For complete cataloguing information, see page 182.

Disclaimer
The recipes in this book have been carefully tested. To the best of our knowledge, they are safe and nutritious for ordinary use and users. All the recipes within this book are gluten-free according to the Canadian Celiac Association dietary guidelines and based on reasonable research for accuracy at the time of writing. For those people with food or other allergies, or who have special food requirements or health issues, please read the suggested contents of each recipe carefully and determine whether or not they may create a problem for you. All recipes are used at the risk of the consumer.

We cannot be responsible for any hazards, loss or damage that may occur as a result of any recipe use.

For those with special needs, allergies, requirements or health problems, in the event of any doubt, please contact your medical adviser prior to the use of any recipe.

Design & Production: PageWave Graphics Inc.
Editor: Sue Sumeraj
Proofreader: Sheila Wawanash
Recipe Tester: Jennifer MacKenzie
Indexer: Belle Wong
Photography: Mark T. Shapiro
Food Stylist: Kate Bush
Props Stylist: Charlene Erricson
Color Scans: Rayment & Collins

Cover image: Apple Pancakes (page 33)

We acknowledge the financial support of the Government of Canada through the Book Publishing Industry Development Program (BPIDP) for our publishing activities.

Published by: Robert Rose Inc.
120 Eglinton Ave. E., Suite 800, Toronto, Ontario, Canada M4P 1E2
Tel: (416) 322-6552 Fax: (416) 322-6936

Printed in Canada
1 2 3 4 5 6 7 8 9 10   FP   14 13 12 11 10 09 08 07 06 05

Contents

Acknowledgements

This book has had the support and assistance of many people from its inception to the final reality.

Our thanks to the following for supplying products for recipe development: Doug Yuen, Dainty Foods, for jasmine and basmati rice, brown rice flour and rice bran; George Birinyi Jr., Grain Process Enterprises Ltd., for arrowroot, potato and tapioca starches, xanthan gum and sorghum, garbanzo-fava, brown rice, chickpea and yellow pea flours; Kingsmill Foods for Egg Replacer®; Diana Phillips and Notta Pasta for rice pasta, St. Dalfour for fruit preserves, including Strawberry, Wild Blueberry and Royal Fig & Pear William, Nakano Rice Vinegars and Caramella Milk Caramel Spread; Jim Grey, Casco, for cornstarch; Danielle Rouleau, Faye Clack Marketing & Communications Inc., for California walnuts and Southern U.S. Trade Association pecans; Connie Priest-Brown, Compass Food Sales, for arrowroot, tapioca and potato starches; Elizabeth and Peter Riesen, El Peto Products Ltd.for rice bran, amaranth, quinoa, sweet rice and flaxseed flours; Michelle Fabian, Nature's Path, for cereals; Maplegrove Foods for Pastariso rice mini-elbows, Mac & Cheese and Pastato potato pasta elbows; Howard Selig, Valley Flaxflour Ltd., for flax flour; Roger Snow for Hemp Hearts®; Greg Herriott, Hempola Inc., for hempseed flour and hemp protein and fiber powder; Richard Abernethy, Canadian Organic Sprout Co., for sprouted flax powder; the employees and owners, The Baker's Catalogue of King Arthur Flour Company, for nut flours, dried fruit, xanthan gum and bread machine yeast; Margaret Hudson, Burnbrae Farms Ltd., for Naturegg Simply Whites; Wendi Hiebert, Ontario Egg Producers, for whole-shell eggs; Michel Dion, Lallamand Inc., for fermipan® yeast; and Joyce Parslow of the Canadian Beef Information Center for sambal oelek.

Thank you to the manufacturers of bread machines who continue to supply the latest models to our test kitchen: Black and Decker and Zojirushi.

A huge thank you to the members of our focus group who faithfully and tirelessly tasted and tested gluten-free recipes and products from beginning to end of recipe development. Thanks to Carol Coulter, Barbara Wahn, Susan Crapper, Sue and Deanna Jennett, Ron Pyatt and Henk Rietveld, and to Lorraine Vinette, RD, Kingston General Hospital, for the nutritional analysis of the Carrot Apple Energy Bars. You'll be pleased to see we listened to and incorporated your suggestions.

We want to express our appreciation to photographer Mark Shapiro, food stylist Kate Bush and prop stylist Charlene Ericson. Thank you for making our gluten-free photographs as delicious-looking as possible. Once again, we enjoyed baking for the photo shoot.

Bob Dees, our publisher, and Marian Jarkovich, Sales and Marketing Manager, National Retail Accounts, at Robert Rose Inc., deserve special thanks for their ongoing support. Thank you to Sue Sumeraj, our editor, and Jennifer MacKenzie, our recipe tester.

To Andrew Smith, Daniella Zanchetta and Joseph Gisini of PageWave Graphics Inc., thank you for working through this cookbook's design, layout and production.

Thank you to our families, husbands, sons, daughters-in-law and grandsons. You helped bring balance to our lives when we became too focused on our work.

And finally, to you, who must follow a gluten-free diet, we sincerely hope these recipes help make your life easier and more enjoyable. We developed them with you in mind.

Introduction

We are excited about this new gluten-free cookbook — our second. Perhaps your family is already enjoying the recipes from our first gluten-free cookbook, *125 Best Gluten-Free Recipes*. We had lots of fun working together (and eating together) on this project, even planning each day's recipe development schedule around lunch. On a typical day, we put a cake in the oven early in the morning, then put a salad dressing in the fridge, mixed muffin batter and simmered soup so all were hot and ready to eat for lunch at one. Our lucky husbands didn't hesitate to share their opinions at dinner.

We continue to bake with sorghum and bean flours, as we are so pleased with the results. Your emails and letters tell us you are sharing the foods you prepare from our baking chapters with the rest of the family. You will notice that we have introduced several new nutritious flours and grains in this book, now that the products are more readily available at grocery and health food stores or through mail order or the web. Quinoa and amaranth — both the grains and the flours — and buckwheat flakes are products that will increase the variety and nutritional value of your diet.

Once again, although you may find a specific combination of flours and starches repeated in several recipes, we have not developed recipes around a "flour mix," but have developed each on its own to give us the taste and baking qualities we desired. This means you'll need to have a greater variety of flours available in your kitchen, and you'll have two or three more measurements to make, but you tell us it is worth it. We *have* included three mixes to save you time. The muffin mix has five variations, the cookie mix has six and the pancake mix has four.

We have met so many terrific people as we take our cookbook to celiac conferences and chapter meetings in both the U.S. and Canada. Thank you for sharing your successes, your recipes and your suggestions for recipes with us. We have adapted several, which are in the book: Macaroni and Cheese, an energy bar, an oil-based pastry and "quick and easy" dinner ideas, just to mention a few. We look forward to meeting you as we travel to introduce this cookbook and share our knowledge and experience at your support group meetings.

Some of our recipes have been inspired by meals we had at restaurants or while traveling. These include a Sticky Date Pudding with Toffee Sauce just like the sticky toffee pudding Donna tasted in a small village in Wales, and a Chocolate Lover's Hazelnut Surprise even better than the volcano cake with a runny chocolate center we shared in a chain restaurant. We have kept up with the latest information on gluten-free ingredients, gluten-free food products and food trends, and we're delighted to pass these tips on to you, along with the easy-to-prepare recipes.

We have tested recipes together for more than ten years, and we still enjoy every bite. As professional home economists, we look at every food from nutritional, food safety and quality angles. We can assure you that every recipe has been tested and tested and tested in our test kitchen. We even researched and purchased new pans, another heavy-duty mixer and several modern kitchen tools, as ours have seen many decades of use and abuse. What a good excuse to re-equip our kitchens!

Celiac friends and focus group members have evaluated the tastes, textures and carrying properties of the baked goods and have prepared the foods to make sure the recipe instructions made sense. We've put the same amount of care and time into this cookbook as we have with our other cookbooks. Check them out by visiting **www.bestbreadrecipes.com**.

We hope you enjoy this collection of gluten-free recipes. Let us know how you and your family enjoy them. We created them just for you!

Donna J. Washburn, PHEc
& Heather L. Butt, PHEc

Quality Professional Services
1655 County Road 2
Mallorytown, Ontario K0E 1R0
or
P.O. Box 1382
Ogdensburg, New York 13669
Phone/Fax: 613-923-2116
Email: **bread@ripnet.com**
Website: **www.bestbreadrecipes.com**

The Gluten-Free Bakeshop Revisited

There is an ever-widening variety of gluten-free flours readily available today in major grocery stores, health food stores and bulk stores, by mail order and on the web.

FLOURS AND STARCHES

We have introduced several new gluten-free flours into our baking repertoire in this cookbook and are enjoying these more nutritious selections. They are fun to work with and lend themselves to tender, delicious products without the gritty texture and starchy aftertaste of some GF products.

The major flours and starches we baked with are described here, and several others are described in the Ingredient Glossary at the back of the book. Unless otherwise specified, store all flours in airtight containers away from heat and light. For more prolonged storage, freeze. They will keep at room temperature for up to 1 month and in the freezer for 1 year.

Amaranth flour is milled from one of the oldest grains, amaranth, called a "super food" by early Aztecs. It is high in protein, fiber, calcium and iron. It has a light, creamy color, a fine texture and a slightly sweet toasted flavor. Store in the refrigerator for up to 1 month. Products high in amaranth may take slightly longer to bake, as it forms a crust on the outside of the product before it is completely baked. Recipes may require less liquid than some other flours.

Arrowroot is the starch made from the roots of a tropical South American plant with large leaves and white flowers. It blends well with all common gluten-free flours. It is referred to as arrowroot starch, as arrowroot flour and as arrowroot starch flour. We use it in berry sauces, as it thickens below the boiling point, giving a warm, clear shine. It must be mixed with a cold liquid before it is added to hot liquids.

Bean flours are high in fiber and calcium, and higher in protein than rice flour. There are several varieties, including garbanzo bean (chickpea), garbanzo-fava (garfava), which combines garbanzo beans and fava beans, and whole bean flour, made from Romano (cranberry) beans. There are both light and dark bean flours: use the dark with chocolate and the light for fruit breads and cakes, or in place of soy flour. Molasses and brown sugar help balance the stronger flavors. Our recipes were developed with whole bean flour, but all bean and pea flours are interchangeable in recipes. Beans are frequently "micronized" to reduce their flatulent effects before being ground to flour. Bean flours can be used in place of rice flour to make cream soups, cream sauces and gravies. Store in the refrigerator for up to 1 month.

Cornstarch is a flavorless, dense white powder from the endosperm of corn. It thickens to a shiny, clear finish, perfect for fruit sauces and glazes. However, cornstarch lumps easily, so it needs to be added to a small amount of cold liquid to make a paste before using. Cornstarch and corn flour are two different products and are not interchangeable.

Nut flour (nut meal) is a flour made by finely grinding nuts such as almonds, hazelnuts or pecans. All nut flours are interchangeable in recipes. Nut flours increase the fiber in a recipe and add a nutty flavor and richness of texture to baked products. Their high fat content aids in browning. Store in the refrigerator for up to 1 month. To make any of the nut flours, see Techniques Glossary, page 181.

Pea flour is high in fiber. It is available in both yellow and green and can be substituted for whole bean flour in baking. Store in the refrigerator for up to 1 month.

Potato starch cannot be interchanged with **potato flour**; they are two distinctly different products. As potato starch lumps easily, sift it before measuring. Potato starch adds moistness to baked goods. Potato flour is too heavy in texture to use in large amounts as a flour substitute in gluten-free recipes.

Quinoa flour is the finely ground cream-colored flour made from the most nutritious grain available. Quinoa (pronounced keen-wah) is the ancient grain of the Incas. It is high in protein, calcium and iron, and is higher in unsaturated fats and lower in carbohydrates than other flours. The grain has a nutty taste and can be eaten as a cereal or used as a rice replacement or a thickener in salads, casseroles or desserts. The small seeds, which look like millet, are naturally coated with a bitter tasting saporin that protects them from birds and insects. Modern processing removes the saporin, and rinsing may not be required (check with the manufacturer). Quinoa flour, used

in small amounts, results in a moist product with good keeping qualities. Store in the refrigerator for up to 1 month.

Rice flour used to be the major flour used in gluten-free baking; however, it cannot be used alone but must be used in combination with starches such as corn, potato or tapioca. The products were frequently gritty, crumbly and dried out quickly. *Brown rice flour* has a grainy texture and provides more fiber than white rice flour. It is a creamy brown in color and we use it in all recipes requiring rice flour. Store in the refrigerator for up to 1 month. *Rice bran and rice polish* are the two outer parts of the rice kernel that have been removed during milling for white rice flour. Rice bran is the outermost layer. When added in small amounts to recipes, they increase the fiber content. Bran and polish are interchangeable in recipes. Store in the refrigerator for up to 1 month to prevent rancidity. *Sweet rice flour* is also known as glutinous rice flour, sticky rice flour or sushi rice flour. It is made from high-starch, sticky short-grain rice, and contains more starch than brown or white rice flour. There are two grades: one is beige, grainy and sandy-textured; the other is white, starchy, sticky and less expensive. The latter works better in recipes. It can be used as a thickener, or to dust baking pans or fingers for easier handling of sticky doughs.

Sorghum flour is made from a millet-like grain, milo (sorghum). It is high in fiber, starch and protein. The round seeds are a little smaller than peppercorns and can be red or white. Rich in fat-soluble and B vitamins, it has a slightly sweet taste; therefore, you are able to decrease the sugar content in recipes with sorghum flour. White sorghum produces flour that is quite white, with tan undertones. Stone-ground sorghum flours brown quickly as they cook. The slightly nutty, savory, very earthy flavor is slightly stronger than that of some gluten-free flours, but used in combination with whole bean flour or amaranth flour, sorghum flour bakes delicious chocolate-, pumpkin- and fig-based treats. We like its thickening properties, and have used it for gravy with success. Sorghum flour is unique, and we have found no substitutes.

Soy flour, high in protein, is a yellow-beige in color and has a slightly nutty flavor. Soy is high in protein, calcium, iron and magnesium. You will notice its strong aroma in a batter, but this disappears when the product is baked. The higher-fat variety browns very quickly, so products may need to be tented with aluminum foil during baking. Store in the refrigerator for up to 1 month.

Tapioca starch (tapioca flour) is a slightly sweet, powdery product made from the cassava root. Use small amounts to sweeten breads made with rice and millet (corn) flours. Sauces require twice the amount of tapioca to thicken as cornstarch, but it continues to thicken as it cools.

Handling Gluten-Free Flours and Starches

- Purchase flours and starches from reliable sources for consistent quality and to ensure that there is no risk from cross-contamination. Once you succeed with a particular product, either brand or quality, stick with it.

- Store flours and starches in plastic containers rather than the bags they are purchased in. Select square, stackable, airtight containers with wide tops and tightly fitting lids to allow for ease of measuring these powdery ingredients.

- Label all containers with easy-to-read permanent markers. It is impossible to tell the difference between some of the white starches by feel or appearance.

- Sift all flours and starches as you fill the containers rather than spending the time each time you bake. Stir with a spoon or fork just before measuring.

- Organize a baking corner where you keep a variety of dry ingredients (store in the refrigerator only those that need to be there). This could be a deep drawer or an overhead cupboard. Keep a set of dry ingredient measures and spoons, a metal spatula, a large metal spoon, a heat-resistant spatula, a set of your most commonly used baking pans and a cooling rack within easy reach.

- Occasionally, you might require a pan previously used for baking a wheat flour recipe. Wash it carefully, as small particles can get trapped in corners. Be especially cautious with pans with ridges, such as the rim of a springform pan.

- Wear a mask if handling gluten-containing flours. They can become airborne, and inhalation can lead to problems.

THICKENING USING
GLUTEN-FREE FLOURS

- Gluten-free flours can be used to thicken gravies, cream sauces, soups and stews when a dull, opaque appearance is desired.

- Either dissolve the GF flour in some cold liquid or cook it in hot fat or drippings for 1 to 3 minutes before adding the remaining cold liquid.

- For more information about thickening with GF flours, see the appendix "Thickener Substitutions" on page 171.

THICKENING USING GLUTEN-FREE STARCHES

- Gluten-free starches can be used to thicken fruit sauces, coulis, custards, Asian food and fruit pies when a clear, glossy appearance is desired.
- Always dissolve the GF starch in cold water, using twice as much liquid as starch, before adding to hot or cold liquids. Liquids may be water, GF stock, milk or juices.
- Do not overcook.
- For more information about thickening with GF starches see the appendix "Thickener Substitutions" on page 171.

Gluten Cross-Contamination in the Kitchen

"Cross-contamination" is the transfer of biological, chemical or physical contaminants to food while processing, preparing, cooking or serving it. Such transfers usually occur when people handle the food. Bacterial cross-contamination can occur when you handle raw then cooked meats, or cut raw meats then vegetables on the same board with the same knife.

If your kitchen is not completely gluten-free, here are a few extra points to help you avoid cross-contamination:

1. Remember, crumbs can hide in silverware and utensil drawers, as well as in baking dishes and cooling racks.

2. Keep a separate cupboard and work area for GF baking supplies and utensils.

3. Purchase a toaster, frying pan, colander, spatula, microwave and bread machine baking pan to use exclusively for GF foods.

4. Purchase and label separate peanut butter, jam, cream cheese and butter to prevent wheat crumbs from contaminating them when a non-GF family member dips in.

5. Purchase squeeze bottles for mustard, GF mayonnaise, relish and GF barbecue sauce.

6. Keep the top shelf in the refrigerator for GF products, so wheat crumbs can't drop in. Be sure to cover all foods in the refrigerator, whether GF or not.

7. If you use a knife block, ensure that all knives are washed well and rinsed before storing. Better yet, keep separate knives and cutting boards for exclusive GF use.

8. Be extra cautious when using wooden cutting boards, and when serving foods in wooden salad bowls, serving dishes or trays.

9. Wipe counters frequently, rinsing and changing cloths between each task to prevent cross-contamination.

Speaking Our Language: Are We All on the Same Page?

1. *"GF" means "gluten-free," such as GF sour cream, GF mayonnaise, etc., when both gluten-free and gluten-containing products are available. We recommend that you read package labels every time you purchase a GF product. Manufacturers frequently change the ingredients.*

2. Our recipes were developed with the following products: large eggs, liquid honey, fancy (not blackstrap) molasses, bread machine (instant) yeast, fruit juice (not fruit drinks), salted butter and 2%, 1% or nonfat milk, yogurt and sour cream (but our recipes will work with other levels of fat). We know you'll get the same great results if you bake with these; expect slightly different results if you make substitutions.

3. Unless otherwise stated in the recipe, eggs and dairy products are used cold from the refrigerator.

4. If the preparation method (chop, melt, dice, slice, etc.) is listed before the food, it means you prepare the food before measuring. If it is listed after the food, measure first, then prepare. Examples are "melted butter" vs. "butter, melted"; "ground flaxseed" vs. "flaxseed, ground"; "cooked brown rice" vs. "brown rice, cooked."

5. Select either metric or imperial measures and stick to one for the whole recipe; do not mix.

6. Use measuring spoons for small amounts. New sets on the market include smidgeon, pinch, dash, $1/8$ tsp, $1/2$ tbsp, 2 tsp and 2 tbsp, in addition to the traditional $1/4$ tsp, $1/2$ tsp, 1 tsp and 1 tbsp. The metric small measures are available in 1 mL, 2 mL, 5 mL, 15 mL and 25 mL sizes. There are also sets of long-handled, narrow spoons made especially to fit into spice jars. These are accurate and fun to use.

7. We use the "spoon lightly into the correct dry measure, heap the top and level once" method of measuring dry ingredients for accuracy and perfect products.

8. Use a graduated, clear liquid measuring cup for all liquids. Place on a flat surface and read at eye level.

9. If in doubt about a food term, a piece of equipment or a specific recipe technique, refer to the glossaries located on pages 172 to 181.

10. All foods that require washing are washed before preparation. Foods such as onion, garlic and bananas are peeled, but fresh peaches and apples are not.

Mixing Methods

Are the terms "cream," "cut in," "fold in" and "whisk" foreign to you? They really are need-to-know terms when you're baking. The wrong speed on the mixer, or an incorrect mixing technique, can result in a completely different product.

Your heavy-duty mixer "use and care" manual will have a chart that explains which numbers or speeds you need to select for the following techniques:

- **Mix, Stir or Combine.** To gently mix ingredients together. (Use the lowest setting or number on the dial.)

- **Cream.** Cookie and cake recipes often begin with "cream the butter and sugar until light and fluffy." Choose the paddle attachment of a heavy-duty electric mixer for the best results. (Use a medium-low setting or number on the dial.)

- **Beat.** This technique usually involves a handheld or heavy-duty electric mixer. (Use a medium-high setting or number on the dial.)
- **Whip**. To beat ingredients vigorously to increase volume and incorporate air. This method typically uses the wire whisk attachment. (Use the highest setting or number on the dial.)

Recipes also often use the following hand techniques:

- **Cut in.** Usually found in biscuit or pastry recipes, this term refers to mixing hard, cold fat with dry ingredients. Choose a special piece of equipment called a pastry blender, or use two knives.

The purpose is to cut the fat into small pieces, coating each small particle with dry ingredients. The resulting dough should be the size of small peas or coarse meal, with some slightly larger pieces. This technique ensures tenderness when the dough is baked.

- **Fold in.** To combine two mixtures of different textures. For example, you fold fruit into whipped cream or GF flours into stiffly beaten egg whites. The tricky part is keeping the air that you have incorporated into the cream or egg whites. Select a large rubber spatula to gently lift and spread the lighter ingredients. Repeat until evenly mixed.
- **Whisk.** To incorporate air quickly, or to blend ingredients in a sauce to prevent it from burning as it cooks. Select a multi-tined wire whisk of a convenient size.

Choosing Baking Pans

- Baking pans are now available in a wide variety of materials: nonstick, aluminum, tin, stainless steel, ceramic and silicone. There are different quality levels of each type. For evenly risen and uniformly browned baked goods, purchase the best quality you can afford.
- We recommend using shiny, light-colored metal pans, as they reflect heat away from the baked product so it doesn't brown too much before it is baked.
- Darker pans absorb more heat and can leave edges crisp and over-browned. When using dark pans, check for doneness 5 minutes before the low end of the recommended baking time. For example, if a recipe says to bake for 35 to 45 minutes, check for doneness after 30 minutes.

- Glass baking dishes and metal baking pans with a nonstick finish conduct and retain heat, causing foods to bake more quickly; therefore, reduce the oven temperature by 25°F (20°C). For example, if a recipe says to bake at 350°F (180°C), bake at 325°F (160°C) instead. When we baked cheesecakes using a dark, nonstick finish, glass-bottomed springform pan, we were much happier with the results we got baking them at the lower temperature.
- For best results, it is important to use the size of pan specifically called for in the recipe.

Rice Cooking Chart

Uncooked rice (1 cup/250 mL)	Amount of liquid*	Cooking time**	Yield	Additional information
White (long-grain)	2 cups (500 mL)	15 minutes	3 cups (750 mL)	
White (medium- or short-grain)	$1\frac{1}{2}$ to $1\frac{3}{4}$ cups (375 to 425 mL)	15 minutes	3 cups (750 mL)	
Brown	2 to $2\frac{1}{2}$ cups (500 to 625 mL)	45 to 50 minutes	3 to 4 cups (750 mL to 1 L)	
Parboiled	2 to $2\frac{1}{2}$ cups (500 to 625 mL)	20 to 25 minutes	3 to 4 cups (750 mL to 1 L)	Also known as converted®. More nutritious than white.
Basmati	2 cups (500 mL)	12 minutes	2 cups (500 mL)	Rinse well before cooking. Let stand, covered, for 5 minutes before serving.
Jasmine	2 cups (500 mL)	15 minutes	2 cups (500 mL)	Rinse well before cooking. Let stand, covered, for 5 minutes before serving.
Wild rice	6 cups (1.5 L)	35 minutes uncovered, then 10 minutes covered	3 cups (750 mL)	Rinse well before cooking. Let stand, covered, for 5 minutes before serving.

* Liquid can be water, GF stock or reconstituted GF stock powder.
** After rice begins to simmer, do not remove the cover and peek. This allows the steam to escape, and the rice can become too dry.

Healthy Choices for Eating Out — or In!

Today, eating out is a challenge for everyone, but even more so for the celiac. You have to worry not only about individual menu items, food preparation methods and cross-contamination in the kitchen, but also about the nutritional content of your selections. To make wise menu choices, follow these suggestions:

1. **Lower-fat or healthy fat items:** Salmon or shellfish, or a stir-fry is always a good choice. Order skim or nonfat milk, ask for GF dressings on the side and remove all visible fat from meat and skin from poultry.

2. **Nutritious choices:** Select dark green salads, roasted vegetables and skim or lower-fat milk rather than mayonnaise-dressed coleslaw, fried vegetables and carbonated beverages. Order a baked potato or a salad instead of french fries (to avoid contamination, ask the wait staff not to cut open the baked potato). Substitute fresh fruit for a heavier dessert.

3. **Method of preparation:** Choose steaming, poaching, grilling and broiling, where individual portions can be prepared on a "super-clean"

(no gluten) surface. Avoid pan-frying, deep-frying and braising, where extra fat is added.

4. **Portion size:** Restaurants use huge serving plates, so keep these serving sizes in mind. Meat should be the same size as a deck of cards. Vegetables should occupy three-quarters of the plate, and each individual vegetable portion should be the size of a computer mouse. Fruit should be the size of a baseball, cheese a 9-volt battery, pasta a tennis ball, and muffins a yo-yo.

5. **Balance:** Don't starve yourself all day and then overeat that evening. Ask for a doggy bag, leave some on your plate or, better yet, ask for a half-portion. Order an appetizer such as steamed mussels as an entrée and share a GF dessert.

Traveling Gluten-Free Safely

More and more families are carrying food from home when they travel by car, plane or train as a result of new, convenient, car-friendly GF foods, the elimination of GF meals on many airlines and the uncertain availability of gluten-free foods along the way. According to a survey by the American Dietetic Association and ConAgra Foods Foundation, 97% of car travelers take food along. Of these, 67% pack sandwiches, 66% take chips and dip, 65% bring fresh fruits and vegetables and 28% pack meat and/or cheese in prepared lunches. Thirty percent leave food unrefrigerated for 3 to 4 hours, and 15% leave food at room temperature for more than 4 hours.*

At home, it is easier to be conscious of food safety and cross-contamination. Remember to follow the same safety rules you follow at home when you're on the road:

1. Wash hands with soap and water for 20 seconds before preparing foods and when switching tasks, such as from handling raw meat, fish or poultry to cutting raw vegetables or from working with wheat products to handling those that are gluten-free.

2. Make sure food preparation areas are clean.

3. Pack moist towelettes so you can wash your hands before eating.

4. Carry perishable food in a cooler containing ice or ice packs. Stow the cooler in the back seat of an air-conditioned car, not the trunk. Include a refrigerator thermometer, and check periodically to make sure the temperature stays below 40°F (4°C). Perishable food left at room temperature for more than an hour is a food safety hazard. If you travel frequently, purchase a cooler that plugs into the cigarette lighter of the car.

5. If stopping along the roadside to grill, watch final cooked temperatures. Hamburgers should reach 160°F (71°C), chicken 170°F (78°F), pork 160°F (71°C) and fish 155°F (68°C). Pack raw meats in the cooler in a well-sealed container separate from other foods.

6. When flying, pack food in small travel cooler bags that fit under an airplane seat. Freeze juice boxes to keep individual insulated lunch bags cool. Freeze bottles of water and drink them as they melt.

7. Carry-out or fast food is also susceptible to food poisoning. If you don't eat or refrigerate it within 2 hours, throw it out. Better yet, refrigerate it promptly.

8. Use the mini-bar refrigerator in your hotel room or ask for an efficiency unit. Request use of the kitchen refrigerator.

* "Beware the En Route Smorgasbord," American Dietetic Association and ConAgra Foods Foundation, March 2004.

Nutritious School Lunches

Between kindergarten and Grade 12, school-children eat approximately 2,400 lunches. Eating healthy meals is equally important for both the celiac and non-celiac child. During the afternoon, students concentrate better and have a higher energy level if they have had a nutritious lunch, resulting in a happier, less stressful learning environment.

Creating healthy, interesting lunches is a constant challenge for every parent. Follow these tasty tips for more nutritious packed lunches:

1. Involve your children in both planning and preparation. They know what is cool to eat. Set some guidelines — one food from each group. Check out the recipes in the box below (see the index for page numbers).

2. Get organized. Keep lunch bags, insulated containers, colorful napkins, plastic cutlery and so forth in one cupboard to make them easy to locate.

3. Insulated lunch bags or boxes are difficult to clean after a day at school, so pack the lunch in a large resealable plastic bag placed inside the lunch container. The plastic bag becomes a lunch box "liner," and washing the lunch box is easier.

When purchasing a new lunch container, consider a soft-sided, aluminum foil–lined one with a removable clear plastic liner held in with Velcro. An ice pack fits nicely between the bag and the clear liner to keep food cold.

4. Send lots of water, juice and milk — enough for both breaks and lunch.

5. Keep cold foods cold. Freeze a juice box to keep eggs, cheese, yogurt, pudding, sandwiches and poultry cold. It thaws by lunch.

6. Keep hot foods hot. Soups and casseroles can be sent in a wide-neck Thermos. Don't forget a spoon!

7. Prevent boredom by sending small treats. Having these prevents children from being tempted to share or trade, as they will be enticed by their own lunch. Remember, treats should be just a small part of the lunch.

8. Consider the nutritive value of the food you pack. Muffins made with carrots, bananas and raisins are better than those made with chocolate chips, and a container of GF trail mix is better than a candy bar.

Bread	Protein	Raw, Raw, Raw	To Quench	Treats
Banana Cranberry Muffins	Mediterranean Pizza Squares	baby carrots and celery sticks	white or chocolate milk	Carrot Apple Energy Bars
Crispy Multi-Seed Crackers	Macaroni and Cheese	red pepper strips and cucumber slices	100% fruit juice	Chocolate Orange Mini-Muffins
Focaccia	Incredibly Easy Pizza Soup	clementines or mandarins	fruit smoothie	Molasses Cookies
Cinnamon Raisin Bread	cream cheese or cheese cubes	apples, grapes or peaches	yogurt shakes	Caramel Apple Cake
Seedy Brown Bread	turkey, tuna, salmon or GF peanut butter	trail mix	water	Pumpkin Date Bars

Grab 'n' Go

Enjoy recipes for a busy lifestyle — quick to prepare, easy to serve, fun to eat!

Cheddar Corn Chowder

Enjoy this delicious chowder by itself for lunch, or add GF ham chunks for a hearty stew.

Tips

Use either a homemade GF chicken stock or reconstitute a commercial GF chicken stock powder.

2 stalks of celery yields ½ cup (125 mL) when sliced.

See Techniques Glossary, page 180, for information about working with fresh herbs.

For a vegetarian version, use GF vegetable stock.

Substitute snipped fresh basil or thyme for the cilantro.

2 tsp	olive oil	10 mL
2	large potatoes, diced	2
2	stalks celery, thinly sliced	2
½	medium onion, diced	½
½	orange bell pepper, diced	½
1 cup	GF chicken stock	250 mL
1	can (14 oz/398 mL) GF cream-style corn	1
1 cup	milk	250 mL
½ cup	frozen corn kernels	125 mL
¼ tsp	dry mustard	1 mL
Pinch	hot pepper flakes	Pinch
¾ cup	shredded old Cheddar cheese, preferably orange-colored	175 mL
2 tbsp to ¼ cup	snipped fresh cilantro	25 to 50 mL
2 tbsp to ¼ cup	snipped fresh parsley	25 to 50 mL
	Salt and freshly ground black pepper	

1. In a large saucepan, heat olive oil over medium heat. Add potatoes, celery, onion and bell pepper; cook for 5 minutes, stirring often. Add stock and bring to a boil. Reduce heat to medium-low and simmer until potatoes are tender, about 15 to 20 minutes.
2. Stir in cream-style corn, milk, frozen corn, dry mustard and hot pepper flakes. Heat gently over medium-low until steaming; do not let boil. Add cheese, cilantro and parsley. Season to taste with salt and pepper. Serve immediately.

Incredibly Easy Pizza Soup

SERVES 4

Don't want all the carbs but crave pizza? Try this version. It will satisfy your cravings.

Tips

Use either a homemade GF beef stock or reconstitute a commercial GF beef stock powder.

2 oz (60 g) fresh mushrooms yield $\frac{1}{2}$ cup (125 mL) sliced.

For 1 cup (250 mL) shredded mozzarella cheese, purchase 4 oz (120 g).

If fresh basil is available, use 2 tbsp (25 mL) chopped.

Substitute cooked hot or mild GF Italian sausage or Italian Sausage Patties (see recipe, page 97) for the pepperoni.

2 tsp	vegetable oil	10 mL
1	small onion, chopped	1
1	clove garlic, minced	1
$\frac{1}{2}$ cup	sliced mushrooms	125 mL
$\frac{1}{4}$ cup	slivered yellow bell pepper	50 mL
1	can (28oz/796 mL) diced tomatoes, with juice	1
5 oz	GF pepperoni, thinly sliced (about 1 cup/250 mL)	150 g
$\frac{1}{2}$ cup	GF beef stock	125 mL
$1\frac{1}{2}$ tsp	dried basil	7 mL
	Salt and freshly ground black pepper	
$\frac{3}{4}$ cup	shredded mozzarella cheese	175 mL
$\frac{1}{4}$ cup	freshly grated Parmesan cheese	50 mL

1. In a large saucepan, heat oil over medium-high heat. Add onion, garlic, mushrooms and yellow pepper. Cook, stirring constantly, until tender, about 5 minutes. Stir in tomatoes, pepperoni, beef stock and basil; bring to a boil. Lower heat to medium-low and simmer for 10 minutes. Season to taste with salt and pepper.

2. Ladle into ovenproof or microwave-safe bowls; sprinkle each with mozzarella and Parmesan. Broil or microwave on High for 45 to 60 seconds, or until cheese melts.

Portobello Mushroom Soup

Be sure to try this intensely flavored modern version of mushroom soup.

Tips

Mushrooms can be stored in a paper bag for up to 3 to 4 days in the refrigerator.

There are 4 portobello mushroom caps in 1 lb (500 g).

The longer and more slowly the mushrooms cook, the fuller the mushroom flavor.

Freeze soup for up to 6 weeks.

1 tbsp	vegetable oil	15 mL
8 oz	Portobello mushrooms (caps sliced, stems whole) (see tip, at left)	250 g
1	onion, coarsely chopped	1
2	cloves garlic, finely chopped	2
1 tbsp	snipped fresh rosemary (or 1 tsp/5 mL dried)	15 mL
¼ tsp	salt	1 mL
¼ tsp	freshly ground white pepper	1 mL
2 tbsp	cornstarch	25 mL
1	can (14 oz/385 mL) 2% evaporated milk	1
1 cup	GF chicken or vegetable stock	250 mL

1. In a large saucepan, heat oil over medium-low heat. Cook mushrooms, onion, garlic, rosemary, salt and pepper, stirring occasionally, for 6 to 8 minutes, or until vegetables are tender but not browned.
2. In a bowl, combine cornstarch, evaporated milk and chicken broth; add to saucepan and bring to a boil, stirring occasionally. Reduce heat to medium-low and simmer for 3 to 4 minutes, or until slightly thickened.
3. Discard mushroom stems. Serve hot.

Variations

Use a variety of mushrooms. Plan to include shiitake, cremini (firmer and with a stronger flavor than a regular white button) and portobellini, as well as portobello (mature cremini with a strong, concentrated flavor).

For a creamy soup, use a food processor to pulse to desired consistency.

For a richer, thicker soup, substitute an equal amount of cream for the evaporated milk.

Broccoli Salad Toss

This versatile all-season salad can be made the day ahead. Be sure to try some of the variations for a different salad every time you make this recipe. Triple this recipe to take to a pot luck, family reunion or company picnic.

Tips

Salad can be made and refrigerated 2 to 3 days in advance. Reserve 1/3 cup (75 mL) of the dressing and add it just before the salad is served.

You can vary the amounts of GF mayo, GF sour cream and yogurt, but keep the total amount at 1 cup (250 mL).

DRESSING

1/3 cup	GF mayonnaise	75 mL
1/3 cup	GF sour cream	75 mL
1/3 cup	plain yogurt	75 mL
2 tbsp	freshly squeezed lemon juice	25 mL

SALAD

1	bunch broccoli, cut into florets (about $6\frac{1}{2}$ cups/1.6 L)	1
8 oz	GF bacon, cooked crisp and crumbled	250 g
1/2 cup	raw unsalted sunflower seeds	125 mL
1/2 cup	raisins	125 mL
2	green onions, sliced	2

1. *Prepare the dressing:* In a small bowl, combine mayonnaise, sour cream, yogurt and lemon juice. Set aside.
2. *Prepare the salad:* In a large bowl, combine broccoli, bacon, sunflower seeds, raisins and green onions. Add dressing and mix well.

Variations

To the basic salad, try adding cauliflower florets, cherry or grape tomatoes, mandarin oranges, feta cheese, red or yellow bell pepper, toasted sesame seeds, toasted slivered almonds, celery or red onions.

Steam broccoli for 1 to 2 minutes; plunge quickly into ice water to stop the cooking.

Baby Spinach Salad with Hot Lemon Dressing

Choose a young, nutritious green leaf to add variety to side salads year round. Increase the number of eggs in the salad to 8 to turn this recipe into 4 main-course lunch salads.

Tips

When preparing leafy greens in advance, wash, dry and then refrigerate, covered with a damp, lint-free tea towel.

Small delicate baby spinach (young spinach) leaves are milder than the mature ones.

Throw out any leftover dressing that was at room temperature for more than 30 minutes.

Today it is recommended that all prepackaged greens be washed again before serving.

SALAD

1	package (10 oz/ 300 g) baby spinach	1
6	slices GF bacon, cooked crisp and crumbled	6
4 oz	sliced mushrooms	125 g
4	hard-cooked eggs, sliced	4
3	thin slices red onion, separated into rings	3

HOT LEMON DRESSING

1/4 cup	butter	50 mL
1	green onion, sliced	1
1 cup	water	250 mL
2 tbsp	sorghum flour	25 mL
2 tbsp	freshly squeezed lemon juice	25 mL
1 tbsp	prepared horseradish	15 mL
1/2 tsp	GF Worcestershire sauce	2 mL
2	hard-cooked eggs, chopped	2

1. *Prepare the salad:* Wash and trim spinach. In a large salad bowl, combine spinach, bacon and sliced mushrooms. Arrange egg slices and onion rings on top.
2. *Prepare the dressing:* In a small saucepan, melt butter over medium heat. Add green onion and cook, stirring, for 1 minute, or until tender. Stir in water, sorghum flour, lemon juice, horseradish and Worcestershire sauce. Bring to a boil, reduce heat to medium-low and simmer for 2 minutes, or until thickened. Stir in eggs. Serve immediately in a small heatproof pitcher alongside spinach salad.

> **Variation**
> Serve the dressing over broiled or grilled salmon or halibut (see recipes, pages 100 and 102).

Cranberry Orange Vinaigrette

The plumped dried cranberries add not only a delightful burst of flavor but also color. Spoon over a mixed green salad topped with a grilled chicken breast.

Tips

Cover and refrigerate for at least 2 hours to allow the flavors to blend and develop. Shake before serving to blend in the oil.

For a better cranberry flavor, choose unsweetened cranberry juice. Avoid drinks, punches or cocktails.

This thick vinaigrette coats the salad; before serving, thin with more orange juice if desired.

1¼ cups	unsweetened cranberry juice	300 mL
¾ cup	freshly squeezed orange juice	175 mL
⅔ cup	dried cranberries	150 mL
2 tbsp	red wine vinegar	25 mL
1 tsp	salt	5 mL
1 tsp	liquid honey	5 mL
1 tsp	Dijon mustard	5 mL
¼ tsp	freshly ground black pepper	1 mL
1 cup	vegetable oil	250 mL

1. In a small saucepan, combine cranberry juice, orange juice, dried cranberries and vinegar. Bring to a boil over medium-high heat. Boil until reduced to 1½ cups (375 mL), about 15 to 20 minutes.
2. Remove from heat and whisk in salt, honey, mustard and pepper. Gradually whisk in oil until blended. Store in a covered jar in the refrigerator for up to 2 weeks.

Variation

For a tangier dressing, double the Dijon mustard and add a clove or two of minced garlic.

Asparagus- and Ham-Filled Crêpes

| MAKES 9 CRÊPES |

Invite your favorite friends for lunch and serve these savory crêpes, hot or cold, topped with corn relish. They'll be a sure hit!

Tips

The crêpes can be made ahead and frozen for up to 1 month. Thaw before filling.

15 to 20 spears of asparagus weigh approximately 1 lb (500 g).

For more information about making crêpes, see page 25.

Substitute GF fruit chutney, GF salsa or Black Bean Salsa (see recipe, page 102) for the corn relish.

6-inch (15 cm) crêpe pan or nonstick skillet, lightly greased

CRÊPES

¼ cup	amaranth flour	50 mL
¼ cup	chickpea (garbanzo bean) flour	50 mL
2 tbsp	potato starch	25 mL
1 tsp	granulated sugar	5 mL
½ tsp	xanthan gum	2 mL
½ tsp	salt	2 mL
½ tsp	dried thyme	2 mL
2	eggs	2
⅔ cup	milk	150 mL
⅓ cup	water	75 mL
1 tbsp	melted butter	15 mL

ASPARAGUS-HAM FILLING

9	slices (each 1 oz/30 g) GF Black Forest ham	9
27	asparagus spears, steamed until just tender-crisp	27
1 cup	corn relish	250 mL

1. *Prepare the crêpes:* In a large bowl, mix together amaranth flour, chickpea flour, potato starch, sugar, xanthan gum, salt and thyme. Set aside.

2. In a small bowl, whisk together eggs, milk, water and melted butter. Pour over dry ingredients all at once and whisk until smooth. Cover and refrigerate for at least 1 hour or for up to 2 days. Bring batter back to room temperature before using.

3. Heat prepared pan over medium heat. Add 3 to 4 tbsp (45 mL to 50 mL) batter for each crêpe, tilting and rotating pan to ensure that batter covers the entire bottom of pan. Cook for 1 to 1½ minutes, or until edges begin to brown. Using a non-metal spatula, carefully turn and cook for another 30 to 45 seconds, or until bottom is dotted with brown spots. Remove to a plate and repeat with remaining batter.

4. *Fill the crêpes:* Place a slice of ham and 3 asparagus spears down the center of each warm crêpe, roll and place seam side down on an individual serving plate.
5. Warm in microwave, if desired. Top with corn relish.

Cooking Classic Crêpes

The secret to making perfect crêpes is simple: practice, practice, practice! In fact, the first crêpe of every batch is just that — a practice one!

- A well-seasoned crêpe pan should be oiled very lightly. Wipe out any excess with a paper towel.
- To test a nonstick crêpe pan or skillet for the correct temperature (375°F/190°C), sprinkle a few drops of cold water on the hot surface. If the water bounces and dances across the pan, it is ready to use. If the water sizzles and evaporates, it is too hot. Adjust the heat if necessary to accomodate differences among cooking utensils and appliances.
- The batter should be smooth and lump-free.
- Set the bowl of batter from the refrigerator directly into a sink of warm water to bring it quickly to room temperature.
- If crêpes stick to pan, cool pan slightly and re-oil. Wipe out any excess with a paper towel — too much oil on pan results in greasy crêpes. Reheat pan before making another crêpe.
- Stack between sheets of parchment or waxed paper as each crêpe is cooked.
- Keep crêpes separated with parchment or waxed paper and store wrapped airtight in the refrigerator for several days or in the freezer for several weeks.
- To prevent tearing, thaw in the refrigerator before separating into individual crêpes.

Garden-Fresh Frittata

A frittata can be described as a Spanish-Italian omelet or a crustless quiche. We cleaned out the refrigerator to prepare this quick and easy any-time-of-day meal.

Tips

See Techniques Glossary, page 180, for information about cleaning leeks, and page 179 for instructions on cleaning a cast-iron skillet.

To ovenproof a nonstick skillet with a non-metal handle, wrap handle in a double layer of foil, shiny side out.

To prevent your cast-iron skillet from rusting, set it on a warm stove element to completely dry before storing. Be careful: the handle gets hot.

Preheat broiler
9- to 10-inch (23 to 25 cm) ovenproof nonstick or cast-iron skillet

1 tbsp	extra-virgin olive oil	15 mL
2	leeks, coarsely chopped, white and light green parts only	2
2	cloves garlic, minced	2
½	red bell pepper, cut into ½-inch (1 cm) cubes	½
2 cups	thickly sliced mushrooms	500 mL
1	small zucchini, cut into ¼-inch (0.5 cm) slices	1
8	egg whites (1 cup/250 mL)	8
4	eggs	4
1 tsp	Dijon mustard	5 mL
¼ cup	snipped fresh chives	50 mL
2 tbsp	snipped fresh parsley	25 mL
2 tsp	dried tarragon	10 mL
½ tsp	salt	2 mL
Pinch	freshly ground white pepper	Pinch
1 cup	broccoli florets, cooked	500 mL
1½ cups	shredded Swiss cheese	375 mL

1. In skillet, heat olive oil over medium heat; add leeks, garlic, red pepper and mushrooms. Cook, stirring frequently, for 5 minutes, or until tender. Add zucchini and cook, stirring, for 2 to 3 minutes, or until vegetables are softened. Remove skillet from heat and reduce heat to medium-low.

2. In a large bowl, whisk together egg whites, eggs, Dijon mustard, chives, parsley, tarragon, salt and pepper. Add broccoli and Swiss cheese, stirring to combine.

3. Pour into skillet over vegetables. Cook, without stirring, for 9 to 11 minutes, or until bottom and sides are firm yet top is still slightly runny.

4. Place under preheated broiler, 3 inches (7.5 cm) from the element, until golden brown and set, 2 to 5 minutes.

5. Cut into wedges and serve hot from the oven or at room temperature. Refrigerate, covered, for up to 2 days. Reheat individual wedges, uncovered, in microwave on Medium (50%) for $1^1/_2$ to 2 minutes, just until hot, if desired.

Variations

For a change from a vegetarian frittata, add cooked chicken, smoked salmon or crisp bacon and use only 1 cup (250 mL) of mushrooms and 1 leek.

Use different varieties of mushrooms for a more intense flavor.

Make-Your-Own Pancake/Waffle Mix

It's great to have this mix on hand when the grandkids come for the weekend. Share some with the adults too! Ron Pyatt emailed a request for a pancake mix recipe, as did the Kingston Chapter of the Canadian Celiac Association for their children's summer camp.

Tips

For added convenience, divide the mix into four portions of 1²/₃ cups (400 mL) each and store in resealable plastic bags. Label and date before storing. We add the page number of the recipe to the label as a quick reference.

Try substituting ¹/₄ cup (50 mL) flaxseed meal for ¹/₄ cup (50 mL) of the almond flour.

1 cup	almond flour	250 mL
1 cup	brown rice flour	250 mL
1 cup	sorghum flour	250 mL
1 cup	soy flour	250 mL
¹/₂ cup	potato starch	125 mL
¹/₂ cup	tapioca starch	125 mL
1 cup	buttermilk powder	250 mL
¹/₃ cup	granulated sugar	75 mL
2 tsp	xanthan gum	10 mL
3 tbsp	GF baking powder	45 mL
1 tbsp	baking soda	15 mL
¹/₂ tsp	salt	2 mL

1. In a very large bowl or a very large plastic bag, combine almond flour, brown rice flour, sorghum flour, soy flour, potato starch, tapioca starch, buttermilk powder, sugar, xanthan gum, baking powder, baking soda and salt. Mix well.

2. Store dry mix in an airtight container in the freezer for up to 6 months. Warm to room temperature before using. Mix well before measuring.

"Small-Batch" Make-Your-Own Pancake/Waffle Mix

Craving pancakes but don't want to make too large a quantity? Use this recipe to make just ten. Great for seniors, singles or hungry teens!

Tips

Recipe can be doubled or tripled.

Use "Small-Batch" in place of ¹/₄ batch Make-Your-Own Pancake/Waffle Mix in the recipes on pages 30 to 33.

¹/₄ cup	almond flour	50 mL
¹/₄ cup	brown rice flour	50 mL
¹/₄ cup	sorghum flour	50 mL
¹/₄ cup	soy flour	50 mL
2 tbsp	potato starch	25 mL
2 tbsp	tapioca starch	25 mL
¹/₄ cup	buttermilk powder	50 mL
2 tbsp	granulated sugar	25 mL
¹/₂ tsp	xanthan gum	2 mL
2¹/₄ tsp	GF baking powder	11 mL
³/₄ tsp	baking soda	4 mL
Pinch	salt	Pinch

1. In a large bowl or plastic bag, combine almond flour, brown rice flour, sorghum flour, soy flour, potato starch, tapioca starch, buttermilk powder, sugar, xanthan gum, baking powder, baking soda and salt. Mix well.
2. Store dry mix in an airtight container in the freezer for up to 6 months. Warm to room temperature before using. Mix well before using.

Plain Jane Waffles

The classic breakfast treat for lazy weekend mornings, these waffles can also be made ahead and enjoyed throughout the week. (See "Pancake/Waffle Know-How," below, for storage tips and reheating instructions.)

Tips

See below for some tips before making waffles.

For a lighter waffle, warm the egg whites before beating (see Techniques Glossary, page 179).

Waffle maker, lightly greased, then preheated

2	eggs, separated	2
¾ cup	water	175 mL
2 tbsp	vegetable oil	25 mL
¼ batch	Make-Your-Own Pancake/Waffle Mix (see recipe, page 28)	¼ batch

1. In a small bowl, using an electric mixer, beat egg whites until stiff but not dry.
2. In a separate bowl, using an electric mixer, beat egg yolks, water and oil until combined. Add waffle mix and beat until smooth. Fold in egg whites.
3. Pour in enough batter to fill preheated waffle maker two-thirds full. Close lid and cook for 6 to 8 minutes, or until no longer steaming. Repeat with remaining batter.

Variation

Add blueberries, chopped apple or nuts to the batter.

Pancake/Waffle Know-How

Preparing gluten-free pancakes differs in several ways from making wheat-based pancakes. Here are some tips from our test kitchen:

- Lightly coat the griddle or nonstick skillet with vegetable oil or cooking spray. Wipe off excess with a paper towel. Dark and light rings on the bottom of pancakes are the result of too much oil on the griddle or skillet.
- To test a nonstick griddle or skillet for the correct temperature (375°F/190°C), sprinkle a few drops of cold water on the hot surface. If the water bounces and dances across the pan, it is ready to use. If the water sizzles and evaporates, it is too hot. Adjust the heat if necessary to accomodate differences among cooking utensils and appliances.
- Resist the temptation to add extra liquid — the batter should be thick.
- Beat the batter until almost smooth — no need to leave it lumpy.

Plain Jane Pancakes

Early spring, and the sap is running. Get ready to make these pancakes. Serve smothered with fresh maple syrup.

Tips

See below for some tips before making pancakes.

Make mini-pancakes for the kids. Be creative and try making panda bear, bunny and happy face shapes.

Griddle or nonstick skillet, lightly greased

2	eggs	2
1	egg white	1
¾ cup	water	175 mL
2 tbsp	vegetable oil	25 mL
¼ batch	Make-Your-Own Pancake/Waffle Mix (see recipe, page 28)	¼ batch

1. In a bowl, using an electric mixer, beat eggs, egg white, water and oil until combined. Add pancake mix and beat until almost smooth.

2. Heat prepared griddle or skillet over medium-high heat. For each pancake, pour ¼ cup (50 mL) batter onto prepared griddle and cook until the bottom is deep golden and the top surface wrinkles around the edges (1 to 3 minutes). Turn and cook for 30 to 60 seconds longer, or until bottom is golden. Serve immediately. Repeat with remaining batter.

- Turn pancakes only once. During development, we kept watching for the bubbles to break before we turned the pancakes. They never did; the top just got wrinkled on the edges. The bottom became deep golden brown, and we were afraid they might burn if cooked any longer before turning. The tops still looked undercooked.
- If pancakes stick to the griddle or skillet, leave them for a few more seconds and try again — they often loosen themselves from the griddle or skillet when it's time to turn them.
- Pancake batter can be refrigerated, covered, for 2 to 3 days. No need to return to room temperature before using.
- Wrap pancakes or waffles well and freeze the extras for up to 1 month. Separate each with a layer of waxed or parchment paper. Reheat frozen pancakes or waffles, straight from the freezer, in either a toaster or a toaster oven.

Blueberry Banana Pancakes

**MAKES ABOUT TEN
4-INCH (10 CM)
PANCAKES**

*Bananas and blueberries
are Donna's grandson
Josh's favorite flavor
combination — and these
pancakes are even better
when served with warm
Blueberry Dessert Sauce
(see recipe, below).*

Tips
Drain thawed frozen
blueberries well to prevent
bleeding into the batter.

See pages 30–31 for
some tips before
making pancakes.

For an all-banana version,
omit the blueberries and
add extra diced banana.

Griddle or nonstick skillet, lightly greased

2	eggs	2
1	egg white	1
1/2 cup	mashed banana	125 mL
1/4 cup	water	50 mL
2 tbsp	vegetable oil	25 mL
1/4 batch	Make-Your-Own Pancake/Waffle Mix (see recipe, page 28)	1/4 batch
2/3 cup	thawed and drained frozen blueberries	150 mL

1. In a bowl, using an electric mixer, beat eggs, egg white, banana, water and oil until combined. Add pancake mix and beat until almost smooth.
2. Heat prepared griddle or skillet over medium-high heat. For each pancake, pour 1/4 cup (50 mL) batter onto prepared griddle. Sprinkle each with 1 to 2 tbsp (15 to 25 mL) blueberries and cook until the bottom is deep golden and the top surface wrinkles around the edges (1 to 3 minutes). Turn and cook for 30 to 60 seconds longer, or until bottom is golden. Serve immediately. Repeat with remaining batter.

Blueberry Dessert Sauce

**MAKES 2 CUPS
(500 mL)**

*Enjoy this versatile
sauce served over
cheesecake, angel food
cake or pancakes.*

1/3 cup	granulated sugar	75 mL
2 tbsp	cornstarch	25 mL
3 cups	frozen blueberries, thawed and drained, juice reserved	750 mL
2 tbsp	freshly squeezed lemon juice	25 mL

1. In a medium saucepan, combine sugar and cornstarch. Slowly add 1/3 cup (75 mL) reserved blueberry juice and lemon juice, stirring constantly. Add blueberries. Cook and stir over medium heat until mixture boils and becomes thick and shiny. Cool, stirring occasionally.

Crispy Pecan Chicken Fingers (page 35)

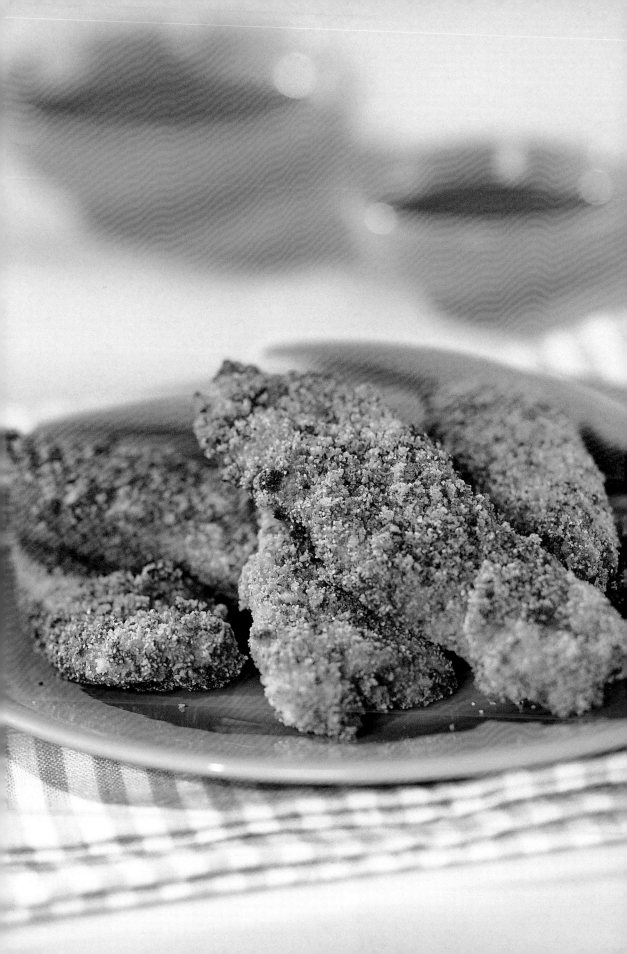

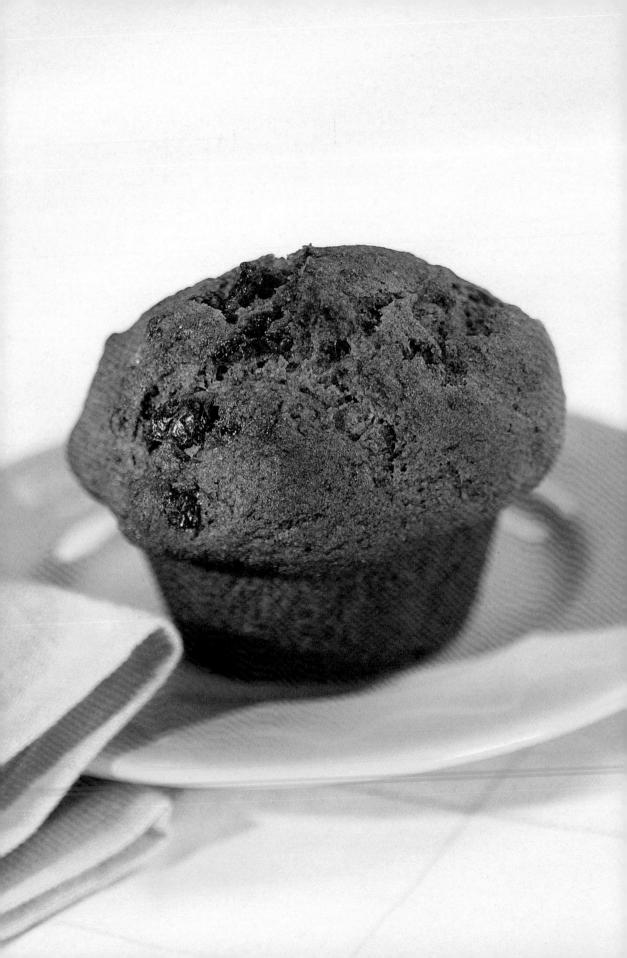

Apple Pancakes

**MAKES ABOUT TEN
4-INCH (10 CM)
PANCAKES**

*A perennial favorite,
apple in the form of
applesauce and chopped
apples contributes the
flavor for these pancakes.*

Tips

Leave the peel on the
apples; the skins soften
as they cook.

See pages 30–31 for
some tips before
making pancakes.

Griddle or nonstick skillet, lightly greased

2	eggs	2
1	egg white	1
¾ cup	unsweetened applesauce	175 mL
¼ cup	water	50 mL
2 tbsp	vegetable oil	25 mL
¼ batch	Make-Your-Own Pancake/Waffle Mix (see recipe, page 28)	¼ batch
1 cup	diced apple	250 mL
1 tsp	ground cinnamon	5 mL

1. In a bowl, using an electric mixer, beat eggs, egg white, applesauce, water and oil until combined. Add the pancake mix, apple and cinnamon and beat until almost smooth.

2. Heat griddle or skillet over medium-high heat. For each pancake, pour ¼ cup (50 mL) batter onto prepared griddle and cook until the bottom is deep golden and the top surface wrinkles around the edges (1 to 3 minutes). Turn and cook for 30 to 60 seconds longer, or until bottom is golden. Serve immediately. Repeat with remaining batter.

Variation

Diced peach, plum or pear or chopped pecans can replace the apple.

Banana Cranberry Muffin
(page 48)

Busy Day Casserole

Barbara Wahn, a local celiac, shared this recipe with us. We modified it for you. Corn, tomato and cheese are a favorite flavor combination from the 50s, still popular today.

Tips

Chili powder may contain gluten; check the label.

Freeze in portion-size pieces to defrost and warm for quick lunches.

Substitute 1 tsp (5 mL) of dried jalapeño pepper for the fresh.

When Barbara makes this casserole, she layers half the cornmeal mixture on the bottom, tops with meat and then finishes with the remaining cornmeal mixture. She also likes to double the recipe so she has lots in the freezer for a busy day.

Substitute extra-lean ground beef for all or part of the ground turkey.

Substitute Monterey Jack or Swiss for all or part of the Cheddar.

Preheat oven to 375°F (190°C)
13- by 9-inch (3 L) baking pan, lightly greased

¾ cup	cornmeal	175 mL
½ cup	milk	125 mL
½ cup	amaranth flour	125 mL
¼ cup	potato starch	50 mL
1 tsp	GF baking powder	5 mL
2 lbs	ground turkey	1 kg
2	cloves garlic, minced	2
1	onion, chopped	1
1	can (28 oz/796 mL) diced tomatoes	1
⅓	jalapeño pepper, chopped	⅓
2 tbsp	GF chili powder	25 mL
2 tbsp	cornstarch	25 mL
2	eggs, beaten	2
1	can (14 oz/398 mL) GF cream-style corn	1
3 tbsp	vegetable oil	45 mL
1 cup	shredded old Cheddar cheese	250 mL
	Black Bean Salsa (see recipe, page 102)	

1. In a small bowl, combine cornmeal and milk. Soak for 20 minutes.
2. In another small bowl, combine the amaranth flour, potato starch and baking powder. Set aside.
3. In a frying pan, over medium heat, brown ground turkey until no pink remains. Add garlic and onion. Cook, stirring, over medium heat until onions are translucent. Drain off fat, if necessary. Add tomatoes, jalapeño pepper, chili powder and cornstarch. Heat until bubbly. Spoon into prepared baking pan.
4. In a large bowl, combine eggs, cream-style corn and oil. Add cornmeal mixture and dry ingredients; stir just until combined. Stir in cheese. Pour over turkey mixture, spreading evenly.
5. Bake in preheated oven for about 35 to 50 minutes, or until a toothpick comes out clean from the cornmeal portion. Serve immediately with Black Bean Salsa.

Crispy Pecan Chicken Fingers

Slender strips of succulent chicken inside a crunchy pecan coating — what a modern, healthier way to eat "fried" chicken! Serve with Plum Dipping Sauce and Honey Mustard Dipping Sauce (see recipes, page 46).

Tips

See Techniques Glossary, page 179, for tips on making fresh bread crumbs.

Shake off excess egg and crumbs before baking.

Chicken is cooked when a digital instant-read thermometer (see Techniques Glossary, page 179) registers 170°F (78°C) and chicken is no longer pink inside.

Discard both leftover crumb mixture and the plastic bag — it is not safe to re-use either when raw chicken is involved.

Preheat oven to 425°F (220°C)
Baking sheet, lightly greased

4	boneless skinless chicken breasts (about 1 lb/500 g)	4
⅓ cup	brown rice flour	75 mL
2	eggs, beaten	2
1 tbsp	water	15 mL
1 tbsp	Dijon mustard	15 mL
1 cup	fresh GF bread crumbs	250 mL
⅔ cup	pecans, coarsely chopped	150 mL
½ cup	cornmeal	125 mL
¼ tsp	salt	1 mL
¼ tsp	freshly ground black pepper	1 mL

1. Cut each breast into strips ³/₄-inch (2 cm) wide. Pat dry.
2. Place the rice flour in a shallow dish or pie plate. In a second shallow dish or pie plate, whisk together eggs, water and Dijon mustard.
3. In a large plastic bag, combine bread crumbs, pecans, cornmeal, salt and pepper.
4. Coat chicken strips, a few at a time, first in rice flour, then in egg mixture. Shake in pecan–bread crumb mixture. Place in a single layer 1 inch (2.5 cm) apart on prepared baking sheet.
5. Bake in preheated oven for 20 to 25 minutes, or until coating is golden brown and crispy and chicken is cooked (see tip, at left).

Variations

Florentine Chicken Fingers: Top baked chicken fingers with grated Asiago cheese, 1 leaf of arugula and a strip of roasted red pepper and broil just until cheese is melted.

Pizza Chicken Fingers: Top baked chicken fingers with GF pizza sauce, grated mozzarella and, if desired, crumbled cooked bacon. Broil just until cheese melts.

Macaroni and Cheese

We received several emails requesting this recipe. We've updated this comfort food from our childhood using 2% evaporated milk and a mixture of cheeses. Martin, Donna's Texas grandson, the family connoisseur of mac and cheese, gives this recipe a "thumbs up."

Tips

Rinsing the cooked pasta well prevents the macaroni and cheese from becoming too thick.

Be sure to use orange-colored Cheddar cheese for a more attractive dish.

We prefer to use wild rice elbow pasta for this recipe.

1 cup	shredded old Cheddar cheese	250 mL
1/2 cup	shredded Swiss cheese	125 mL
1/4 cup	freshly grated Parmesan cheese	50 mL
1 tbsp	sorghum flour	15 mL
1/2 tsp	dry mustard	2 mL
1/2 tsp	salt	2 mL
1/4 tsp	freshly ground white pepper	1 mL
Pinch	cayenne pepper	Pinch
2 cups	GF elbow pasta	500 mL
1	can (14 oz/385 mL) 2% evaporated milk	1
1/4 tsp	GF Worcestershire sauce	1 mL

1. In a small bowl, combine Cheddar, Swiss, Parmesan, sorghum flour, dry mustard, salt, white pepper and cayenne pepper. Set aside.
2. In a large saucepan, cook pasta in boiling water according to package instructions, until just tender. Rinse well under cold running water and drain well.
3. Return the pasta to the saucepan. Stir in milk, Worcestershire sauce and cheese mixture. Simmer, stirring gently, over low heat until mixture boils and thickens.

Variation

To turn this into a casserole, add canned tuna, peas and chopped onion or celery, transfer to a greased baking dish and bake in preheated 350°F (180°C) oven until hot.

Cheddar Dill Shortbread

A new twist on an old familiar favorite — turn a traditional sweet, rich cookie into a savory melt-in-your-mouth hors d'oeuvre.

Tips

Select white Cheddar for a more traditional shortbread appearance.

If dough appears too soft, don't add extra flour. Instead, using the waxed paper, form into a log. Then refrigerate just until firm, slice and bake.

If you want to make cookies another day, store the dough logs in the refrigerator for up to 1 week. Let stand at room temperature for 45 minutes to 1 hour before slicing and baking.

For longer storage of the dough logs, freeze for up to 2 months. Defrost in the refrigerator overnight and then let stand at room temperature for 45 minutes to 1 hour before slicing and baking.

Preheat oven to 350°F (180°C)
Baking sheet, ungreased

1 cup	shredded old Cheddar cheese	250 mL
¾ cup	butter, softened	175 mL
½ cup	rice flour	125 mL
⅓ cup	cornstarch	75 mL
¼ cup	potato starch	50 mL
2 tbsp	tapioca starch	25 mL
⅓ cup	sifted confectioner's (icing) sugar	75 mL
¼ cup	freshly grated Parmesan cheese	50 mL
1 to 2 tbsp	finely chopped fresh dill	15 to 25 mL

1. In a food processor fitted with a metal blade, pulse Cheddar, butter, rice flour, cornstarch, potato starch, tapioca starch, confectioner's sugar, Parmesan and dillweed to taste until mixed. Process until dough forms a ball.

2. Place dough on waxed paper, form into logs 1½ inches (4 cm) in diameter, and wrap tightly. Refrigerate for at least 2 hours, or until firm. Cut into slices ¼ inch (0.5 cm) thick. Place 1 inch (2.5 cm) apart on baking sheet. Bake in preheated oven for 8 to 12 minutes, or until set but not browned. Remove immediately from baking sheet to cooling rack. Serve warm or at room temperature.

Variation

Omit the dillweed and add a pinch of cayenne pepper or 1 to 2 tbsp (15 to 25 mL) GF curry powder.

Mediterranean Pizza Squares

Try our twist on a traditional pizza crust. This vegetarian pizza, with an easy-to-prepare crust, is delicious served hot or at room temperature for a snack, lunch or brunch.

Tips

See Techniques Glossary, page 180 for instructions on roasting garlic.

This is a very thin crust. There is enough dough to cover the bottom of the pan evenly with a thin layer. Take your time.

For fast, easy cutting, use a pizza wheel.

Cut into 48 bite-size appetizers for your next party.

Substitute mozzarella, fontina or provolone cheese for the Monterey Jack.

Preheat oven to 425°F (220°C)
15- by 10-inch (40 by 25 cm) jelly-roll pan, lightly greased and sprinkled with cornmeal

1 cup	amaranth flour	250 mL
1/2 cup	quinoa flour	125 mL
1/4 cup	cornstarch	50 mL
1/4 cup	cornmeal	50 mL
1 tsp	xanthan gum	5 mL
1 tbsp	GF baking powder	15 mL
1 tsp	salt	5 mL
1/3 cup	shortening	75 mL
3/4 cup	milk	175 mL
	Sweet rice flour	
3	plum tomatoes, thinly sliced	3
4	cloves garlic, roasted and chopped	4
2/3 cup	sliced black olives	150 mL
1/4 cup	snipped fresh basil	50 mL
1/4 tsp	freshly ground black pepper	1 mL
1 cup	shredded Monterey Jack cheese	250 mL
1 cup	crumbled feta cheese	250 mL

Traditional Method

1. In a large bowl, stir together amaranth flour, quinoa flour, cornstarch, cornmeal, xanthan gum, baking powder and salt. Using a pastry blender or two knives, cut in shortening until mixture resembles coarse crumbs. Add milk, all at once, stirring with a fork to make a soft dough.

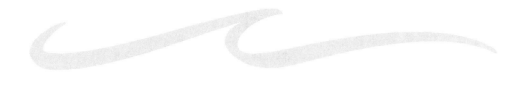

Substitute an equal amount of chopped fresh rosemary for the basil.

To make the pizza kid-friendly, top with their favorite fixings. Keep one in the freezer for when they are invited to a pizza party.

Food Processor Method

1. In a food processor fitted with a metal blade, pulse amaranth flour, quinoa flour, cornstarch, cornmeal, xanthan gum, baking powder and salt. Add shortening and pulse until mixture resembles small peas, about 5 to 10 seconds. With the machine running, pour milk through feed tube and process until dough just holds together.

For Both Methods

2. Transfer dough to prepared pan. Either cover with waxed paper and roll out with a rolling pin or gently pat out dough with fingers dusted with sweet rice flour to fill the pan evenly. Bake in the bottom third of preheated oven for 10 minutes or until slightly firm.

3. Arrange tomato slices over crust; sprinkle with garlic, olives, basil and pepper. Sprinkle with Monterey Jack and feta.

4. Bake in preheated oven for 20 to 25 minutes, or until cheese is bubbly and crust is golden. Remove to a cutting board and cut into squares. Serve immediately. Transfer any extra squares to a cooling rack to prevent the crust from getting soggy.

Crispy-Coated Veggie Snacks

These healthier crispy baked tidbits are an appealing alternative to deep-fried fare.

Tips

For information on making dry bread crumbs, see Techniques Glossary, page 179.

Serve with salsa, Broccoli Cilantro Pesto (see recipe, page 96), GF sour cream or your favorite dipping sauce.

Use other vegetables, such as cauliflower, broccoli or white turnip.

Use any leftover savory bread, such as Italian Herb Bread (see recipe, pages 70–71) or Southern Cornbread (see recipe, page 64) to make the bread crumbs.

Preheat oven to 375°F (190°C)
Baking sheet, lightly greased

1	small zucchini	1
1	small sweet potato	1
12	small mushrooms	12
3 cups	dry GF bread crumbs	750 mL
1 cup	freshly grated Parmesan cheese	250 mL
1 tbsp	dried rosemary or thyme	15 mL
Pinch	cayenne pepper	Pinch
2 cups	plain yogurt	500 mL
	Honey Mustard Dipping Sauce or Plum Dipping Sauce (see recipes, page 46)	

1. Peel zucchini, cut in half crosswise and cut each half lengthwise into quarters.
2. Peel sweet potato, cut in half lengthwise and cut into slices 1/4 inch (0.5 cm) thick.
3. Remove stems from mushrooms.
4. In a shallow dish or pie plate, combine bread crumbs, Parmesan cheese, rosemary and cayenne pepper.
5. Working with a few pieces at a time, dip zucchini, sweet potato and mushroom caps into yogurt to generously coat. Then dip into crumb mixture, pressing to coat well.
6. Arrange on prepared baking sheet in a single layer. Bake in preheated oven for 20 to 25 minutes, or until vegetables are tender and coating is golden.
7. Transfer to a serving plate and serve immediately with Honey Mustard Dipping Sauce or Plum Dipping Sauce.

Baked Mozzarella Sticks

MAKES 12

Crave mozzarella sticks but don't want to deep-fry? These crispy baked sticks are worth the extra care.

Tips

For information on making dry bread crumbs, see Techniques Glossary, page 179.

To prevent melted cheese from leaking out, be sure each piece is completely coated with yogurt mixture and crumbs.

Serve with salsa, Broccoli Cilantro Pesto (see recipe, page 96), GF sour cream or your favorite dipping sauce.

To freeze: Double or triple the recipe and freeze coated unbaked cheese sticks in a single layer in a jelly-roll pan. Once frozen, remove cheese sticks from pan and place in a heavy-duty freezer bag. Remove only the number you need — they won't stick together. Bake according to recipe.

Use any leftover savory bread, such as Italian Herb Bread (see recipe, pages 70–71) or Southern Cornbread (see recipe, page 64) to make the extra-fine bread crumbs.

Preheat oven to 450°F (230°C)
Baking sheet, lightly greased

8 oz	mozzarella cheese	250 g
2	egg yolks	2
1 cup	plain yogurt	250 mL
2 cups	extra-fine dry GF bread crumbs	500 mL
$2/3$ cup	freshly grated Parmesan cheese	150 mL
1 tbsp	dried basil or dillweed	15 mL
Pinch	cayenne pepper	Pinch

1. Cut mozzarella cheese into sticks 3 by $1/2$ by $1/2$ inch (7.5 by 1 by 1 cm).
2. In a small bowl, combine egg yolks and yogurt.
3. In a shallow dish or pie plate, combine bread crumbs, Parmesan, basil and cayenne pepper.
4. Dip cheese into yogurt-mixture to generously coat, leaving as much mixture on the cheese as possible. Then dip into crumb mixture, pressing to coat ends and sides well.
5. Place the coated sticks in a single layer on prepared baking sheet and freeze for 2 to 4 hours, or until completely frozen. Bake in preheated oven for 5 to 8 minutes, or until coating is golden.
6. Transfer to a serving plate and serve immediately.

Crispy Multi-Seed Crackers

*Whether being dipped
in salsa or served with
a bowl of hot soup, these
crisp, Lavosh-style crackers
will add heart-healthy
omega-3 fatty acids and
fiber to your diet.*

Tips
Buy flaxseed already
ground or grind your own
in a clean coffee grinder.

For a thin crisp cracker,
roll dough to an even
thickness as thinly as
possible. Don't worry if
it breaks into pieces.

Pay close attention
during the last few
minutes of baking, as
crackers can burn easily.

If crackers become soft,
re-crisp in a toaster oven
or conventional oven at
350°F (180°C).

Just before baking,
sprinkle with 1 tsp
(5 mL) coarse salt or
sesame seeds.

Substitute an equal
amount of hempseed
flour for the ground
flaxseed.

Preheat oven to 375°F (190°C)
Baking sheets, ungreased

½ cup	water	125 mL
2 tbsp	extra-virgin olive oil	25 mL
1 tsp	cider vinegar	5 mL
½ cup	brown rice flour	125 mL
½ cup	sorghum flour	125 mL
¼ cup	cornstarch	50 mL
⅓ cup	ground flaxseed	75 mL
1½ tsp	xanthan gum	7 mL
½ tsp	GF baking powder	2 mL
1 tsp	salt	5 mL
¼ cup	freshly grated Parmesan cheese	50 mL
¼ cup	sesame seeds	50 mL
3 tbsp	dried oregano	45 mL
2 tbsp	poppy seeds	25 mL

1. In a small bowl, combine water, olive oil and vinegar.
   Mix well and set aside.

2. In a food processor fitted with a metal blade, pulse brown
   rice flour, sorghum flour, cornstarch, ground flaxseed,
   xanthan gum, baking powder, salt, Parmesan, sesame
   seeds, oregano and poppy seeds until mixed. With
   machine running, add liquid mixture through feed tube
   in a slow steady stream. Process until dough forms a ball.

3. Divide dough into four pieces. Place each on plastic
   wrap and flatten into a disk; wrap well. Let dough rest
   in refrigerator for 10 minutes. Place one disk between
   two sheets of waxed or parchment paper. To prevent
   the paper from moving while you're rolling out the
   dough, place it on a lint-free towel. Using a heavy
   stroke with a rolling pin, roll out the dough as thinly
   as possible. Carefully remove the top sheet of paper.
   Invert the dough onto the baking sheet. Remove
   remaining sheet of paper. Repeat with remaining dough.

4. Bake in preheated oven for 18 to 25 minutes, or until
   browned and crisp. Remove to a cooling rack and cool
   completely. Break into pieces. Store at room temperature
   in an airtight container for up to 2 weeks or freeze for
   up to 3 months.

Carrot Apple Energy Bars

MAKES 18 BARS

For a quick, easy, on-the-move breakfast or snack, choose these moist, nutritious bars. Lorraine Vinette, RD, a dietitian at Kingston General Hospital provided the nutritional analysis.

Tips

When cut into eighteen 3- by 2-inch (7.5 by 5 cm) bars, each contains 172 calories, 7 grams of protein, 31 grams of carbohydrates, 4.4 grams of fat and 3.6 grams of fiber.

For the dried fruit mix, we used ¼ cup (50 mL) dried cranberries, ¼ cup (50 mL) raisins, 2 tbsp (25 mL) dried mangoes, 1 tbsp (15 mL) dried blueberries and 1 tbsp (15 mL) dried apricots.

Check for gluten if you purchase the fruit as a prepared mix.

For a lactose-free bar, omit the milk powder.

Try substituting grated zucchini for all or half of the carrots.

Substitute cardamom for the cinnamon.

Preheat oven to 325°F (160°C)
13- by 9-inch (3 L) baking pan, lined with foil and lightly greased

1¼ cups	sorghum flour	300 mL
½ cup	amaranth flour	125 mL
⅓ cup	rice bran	75 mL
¼ cup	ground flaxseed	50 mL
½ cup	nonfat (skim) milk powder	125 mL
1½ tsp	xanthan gum	7 mL
1 tbsp	GF baking powder	15 mL
¼ tsp	salt	1 mL
2 tsp	ground cinnamon	10 mL
2	eggs	2
1 cup	unsweetened applesauce	250 mL
⅓ cup	packed brown sugar	75 mL
1½ cups	grated carrots	375 mL
¾ cup	dried fruit mix (see tips, at left)	175 mL
½ cup	chopped walnuts	125 mL

1. In a large bowl or plastic bag, combine sorghum flour, amaranth flour, rice bran, ground flaxseed, milk powder, xanthan gum, baking powder, salt and cinnamon. Mix well and set aside.

2. In a separate bowl, using an electric mixer, beat eggs, applesauce and brown sugar until combined.

3. Add flour mixture and mix just until combined. Stir in carrots, dried fruit and nuts. Spoon into prepared pan, spread to edges with a moist rubber spatula and allow to stand for 30 minutes.

4. Bake in preheated oven for 30 to 35 minutes, or until a cake tester inserted in the center comes out clean. Let cool in pan on a cooling rack and cut into bars. Store in an airtight container at room temperature for up to 1 week or individually wrapped and frozen for up to 1 month.

Linda's Granola

Every time you make this granola, challenge yourself to add variety by trying coconut, soy nuts, walnuts, pistachios, macadamia nuts, pecans, buckwheat flakes, apricots, dates, dried apple slices, blueberries and pineapple. Serve for breakfast, as a snack or as a nibble on your next hike.

Tips

For the GF multigrain cereal, we used a purchased boxed cereal with a mixture of corn, flaxseeds, amaranth and quinoa.

For the mixed dried fruit, we used a mixture of banana slices, papaya, raisins and cranberries. Vary the mix of dried fruit and the kind of nuts; just keep the total volume at 4 cups (1 L).

Substitute an equal amount of liquid honey for the corn syrup.

For the GF multigrain cereal, substitute GF puffed rice.

Spray the large stirring spoon with cooking spray to prevent sticking.

Preheat oven to 300°F (150°C)
Two 15- by 10-inch (40 by 25 cm) jelly-roll pans, lightly greased

½ cup	corn syrup	125 mL
1 tbsp	vegetable oil	15 mL
4 cups	GF multigrain cereal	1 L
2 cups	GF honeyed corn flakes cereal	500 mL
1 cup	mixed nuts	250 mL
1 cup	whole almonds	250 mL
½ cup	sunflower seeds	125 mL
½ cup	pumpkin seeds	125 mL
3 cups	mixed dried fruit	750 mL

1. In a glass measuring cup, combine corn syrup and oil. Microwave, uncovered, on High for 45 seconds, or until it can be easily poured.

2. In a very large bowl, combine multigrain cereal, corn flakes cereal, mixed nuts, almonds, sunflower seeds and pumpkin seeds. Pour in corn syrup mixture and stir to coat evenly. Spread in prepared pans.

3. Bake in preheated oven for 30 to 40 minutes, or until toasted, stirring every 10 minutes. Add dried fruit. Stir gently to combine. Bake for 10 minutes more. Let cool in oven for 1 hour, with the oven turned off. Let cool completely on pans on a cooling rack. Store at room temperature in airtight containers for up to 3 months.

Garlic Bean Dip

Cannellini beans are popular in Italy. Their creamy color, fluffy texture and mild, nutty taste blends well in this garlic-flavored bean dip.

Tips

Serve at either room temperature or straight from the refrigerator with Crispy Multi-Seed Crackers (see recipe, page 42).

Rinse and drain beans well to ensure a consistent thickness of dip each time you make it.

Substitute chickpeas (garbanzo beans) for the cannellini beans *or* one 19-oz (540 mL) can of Bean Medley *or* one 19-oz (540 mL) can of 6-Bean Blend.

For a tangier flavor, substitute plain yogurt or GF sour cream for the mayonnaise.

2	cloves garlic, minced	2
1	can (19 oz/540 mL) cannellini or white kidney beans, rinsed and drained	1
1 tbsp	cider vinegar	15 mL
½ tsp	salt	2 mL
½ tsp	ground cumin	2 mL
⅓ cup	GF light mayonnaise	75 mL
2 tbsp	fresh parsley	25 mL

1. In a food processor fitted with a metal blade, pulse garlic, beans, vinegar, salt and cumin until mixed. Add mayonnaise and parsley and process until smooth. Transfer to a bowl, cover and refrigerate for at least 6 hours or overnight to allow flavors to mix and mingle. Refrigerate for up to 1 week.

Honey Mustard Dipping Sauce

¼ cup	Dijon mustard	50 mL
¼ cup	liquid honey	50 mL

1. In a small bowl, combine Dijon mustard and honey. Serve at room temperature. (If the honey becomes too thick to pour, microwave, uncovered, on Medium (50%) for a few seconds until it pours easily.)

"Grandma, you make the best sauce in the whole wide world — please make more," declares Donna's grandson Andrew, holding up the last two Crispy Pecan Chicken Fingers (see recipe, page 35).

Variation
Substitute prepared or grainy mustard for the Dijon.

Plum Dipping Sauce

MAKES 1 CUP (250 mL)

1	can (14 oz/398 mL) prune plums	1
⅓ cup	granulated sugar	75 mL
3 tbsp	vinegar	45 mL

1. Drain plums, reserving 2 tbsp (25 mL) liquid. Remove pits from plums. In a blender, purée plums and reserved liquid.
2. In a small saucepan, combine plum purée, sugar and vinegar. Heat over medium heat until mixture comes to a gentle boil. Remove from heat and let cool before serving.

Try this quick and easy, rich plum-colored sauce with Crispy Pecan Chicken Fingers (see recipe, page 35) for your next kids' party. Save some for the adults too!

Tips

Sauce can be stored, covered, in the refrigerator for up to 2 weeks.

To prevent cross-contamination, set out individual bowls for dipping sauces for each person.

Serve sauce warm or cold — it's delicious either way!

Variations
In season, 8 fresh plums can be substituted for the canned plums. For an even quicker sauce, substitute one 7.5-oz (213 mL) jar of GF baby food strained plums.

To add tomato flavor, add 1 tbsp (15 mL) GF ketchup or GF barbecue sauce to the dipping sauce.

Muffins, Loaves and More

Hot from the oven for a weekend breakfast, or packed frozen for lunch, these quick breads are too delicious to resist.

Banana Cranberry Muffins or Loaf

MAKES 12 MUFFINS OR 1 LOAF

Bake extras to store in the freezer for those mornings when you're running late. Everybody loves to grab a muffin, and add a chunk of cheese and an apple for a quick on-the-run breakfast.

Tips

If muffins stick to the pan, let stand for 2 to 3 minutes, then try again to remove them.

Use an ice cream scoop to portion an even amount of batter into each muffin cup.

For a tangier flavor, replace dried cranberries with fresh or frozen.

You can substitute strawberry-, orange- or cherry-flavored dried cranberries.

If quinoa flour is not available, substitute an equal amount of brown rice flour.

12-cup muffin tin or 9- by 5-inch (2 L) loaf pan, lightly greased

1 cup	sorghum flour	250 mL
1/3 cup	quinoa flour	75 mL
1/3 cup	tapioca starch	75 mL
1/2 cup	granulated sugar	125 mL
1 tsp	xanthan gum	5 mL
1 tbsp	GF baking powder	15 mL
1 tsp	baking soda	5 mL
1/4 tsp	salt	1 mL
2	eggs	2
1 1/4 cups	mashed banana (about 3)	300 mL
1/4 cup	vegetable oil	50 mL
1 tsp	cider vinegar	5 mL
3/4 cup	dried cranberries	175 mL

1. In a large bowl or plastic bag, combine sorghum flour, quinoa flour, tapioca starch, sugar, xanthan gum, baking powder, baking soda and salt. Mix well and set aside.
2. In a separate bowl, using an electric mixer, beat eggs, banana, oil and vinegar until combined. Add dry ingredients and mix just until combined. Stir in cranberries.

For Muffins
3. Spoon batter evenly into each cup of prepared muffin tin. Let stand for 30 minutes. Meanwhile, preheat oven to 350°F (180°C). Bake in preheated oven for 18 to 20 minutes, or until firm to the touch. Remove from the pan immediately and let cool completely on a rack.

For a Loaf
3. Spoon batter into prepared loaf pan. Let stand for 30 minutes. Meanwhile, preheat oven to 350°F (180°C). Bake in preheated oven for 55 to 65 minutes, or until a cake tester inserted in the center comes out clean. Let cool in the pan on a rack for 10 minutes. Remove from the pan and let cool completely on a rack.

Blueberry Orange Muffins or Loaf

If you enjoy blueberries, you'll love the intriguing flavor of this speckled orange treat.

Tips

Mix the dry ingredients thoroughly before adding to the liquids; the gluten-free flours and starch are so finely textured they clump very easily.

Using dried blueberries ensures that this breakfast bread or teatime snack doesn't have a bluish tinge, as it would with fresh or frozen blueberries.

As soon as muffins cool to room temperature, wrap individually in plastic wrap and freeze for up to 1 month for a grab-and-go breakfast or lunch.

For special occasions, sprinkle 2 tbsp (25 mL) sliced almonds and 1 tbsp (15 mL) granulated sugar over the top just before baking.

12-cup muffin tin or 9- by 5-inch (2 L) loaf pan, lightly greased

1¼ cups	amaranth flour	300 mL
½ cup	brown rice flour	125 mL
⅓ cup	tapioca starch	75 mL
½ cup	granulated sugar	125 mL
1½ tsp	xanthan gum	7 mL
1 tbsp	GF baking powder	15 mL
½ tsp	salt	2 mL
2	eggs	2
1 tbsp	grated orange zest	15 mL
1 cup	freshly squeezed orange juice	250 mL
2 tbsp	vegetable oil	25 mL
½ cup	slivered almonds	125 mL
½ cup	dried blueberries or cranberries (see tip, at left)	125 mL

1. In a large bowl or plastic bag, combine amaranth flour, brown rice flour, tapioca starch, sugar, xanthan gum, baking powder and salt. Mix well and set aside.
2. In a separate bowl, using an electric mixer, beat eggs, orange zest, orange juice and oil until combined. Add dry ingredients and mix just until combined. Fold in almonds and blueberries.

For Muffins

3. Spoon batter evenly into each cup of prepared muffin tin. Let stand for 30 minutes. Meanwhile, preheat oven to 350°F (180°C). Bake in preheated oven for 18 to 20 minutes, or until firm to the touch. Remove from the pan immediately and let cool completely on a rack.

For a Loaf

3. Spoon batter into prepared loaf pan. Let stand for 30 minutes. Meanwhile, preheat oven to 350°F (180°C). Bake in preheated oven for 55 to 65 minutes, or until a cake tester inserted in the center comes out clean. Let cool in the pan on a rack for 10 minutes. Remove from the pan and let cool completely on a rack.

Figgy Apple Muffins or Loaf

MAKES 12 MUFFINS OR 1 LOAF

Never baked with figs before but always wanted to try them? Bake these moist, not-too-sweet muffins that are sure to please everyone.

Tips

Make your own applesauce: just slice and core the apples, blend in a blender and sweeten to taste. No need to peel the apples or cook them.

This is a very dark loaf, depending on the type of pan used; you may want to lower the oven temperature by 25°F (20°C).

Substitute ¾ cup (175 mL) chopped apple for the applesauce and ½ cup (125 mL) commercial fig spread for the chopped dried figs. We found that a fig spread sweetened with only grape juice concentrate worked perfectly in this recipe.

12-cup muffin tin or 9- by 5-inch (2 L) loaf pan, lightly greased

1¼ cups	sorghum flour	300 mL
⅓ cup	whole bean flour	75 mL
¼ cup	cornstarch	50 mL
¼ cup	rice bran	50 mL
⅓ cup	granulated sugar	75 mL
1½ tsp	xanthan gum	7 mL
1 tbsp	GF baking powder	15 mL
¼ tsp	salt	1 mL
1 tsp	ground cardamom	5 mL
2	eggs	2
1 cup	plain yogurt	250 mL
½ cup	sweetened applesauce	125 mL
¼ cup	vegetable oil	50 mL
1 tsp	cider vinegar	5 mL
¾ cup	chopped dried figs	175 mL

1. In a large bowl or plastic bag, combine sorghum flour, whole bean flour, cornstarch, rice bran, sugar, xanthan gum, baking powder, salt and cardamom. Mix well and set aside.

2. In a separate bowl, using an electric mixer, beat eggs, yogurt, applesauce, oil and vinegar until combined. Add dry ingredients and mix just until combined. Stir in figs.

For Muffins

3. Spoon batter evenly into each cup of prepared muffin tin. Let stand for 30 minutes. Meanwhile, preheat oven to 350°F (180°C). Bake in preheated oven for 18 to 23 minutes, or until firm to the touch. Remove from the pan immediately and let cool completely on a rack.

For a Loaf

3. Spoon batter into prepared loaf pan. Let stand for 30 minutes. Meanwhile, preheat oven to 350°F (180°C). Bake in preheated oven for 55 to 65 minutes, or until a cake tester inserted in the center comes out clean. Let cool in the pan on a rack for 10 minutes. Remove from the pan and let cool completely on a rack.

Pecan Pear Muffins or Loaf

Delicately flavored pears provide both moistness and fiber. Enjoy with dark grapes and a wedge of ripe Camembert, Boursin or Brie.

Tips

No need to peel the pears — the skins soften during baking.

For best results, fruit should be perfectly ripe. If necessary, ripen fruit in a paper bag on the counter until it is fragrant and yields to gentle thumb pressure near the base of the stem. Check daily — it may take anywhere from 1 to 8 days.

For each 1 cup (250 mL) of coarsely chopped pear, purchase one large Anjou or Bartlett pear.

Substitute a 7½-oz (225 mL) jar of commercial pear spread for the chopped pears. We found that a pear spread sweetened with only grape juice concentrate worked perfectly in this recipe.

12-cup muffin tin or 9- by 5-inch (2 L) loaf pan, lightly greased

1 cup	sorghum flour	250 mL
¼ cup	quinoa flour	50 mL
¼ cup	potato starch	50 mL
½ cup	granulated sugar	125 mL
1½ tsp	xanthan gum	7 mL
1 tbsp	GF baking powder	15 mL
½ tsp	salt	2 mL
1 tsp	ground ginger	5 mL
2	eggs	2
¾ cup	plain yogurt	175 mL
¼ cup	vegetable oil	50 mL
2 tsp	grated lemon zest	10 mL
2 tsp	freshly squeezed lemon juice	10 mL
1½ cups	coarsely chopped pears	375 mL
⅔ cup	coarsely chopped pecans	150 mL

1. In a large bowl or plastic bag, combine sorghum flour, quinoa flour, potato starch, sugar, xanthan gum, baking powder, salt and ginger. Mix well and set aside.
2. In a separate bowl, using an electric mixer, beat eggs, yogurt, oil, lemon zest and lemon juice until combined. Add dry ingredients and mix just until combined. Stir in pears and pecans.

For Muffins
3. Spoon batter evenly into each cup of prepared muffin tin. Let stand for 30 minutes. Meanwhile, preheat oven to 350°F (180°C). Bake in preheated oven for 18 to 20 minutes, or until firm to the touch. Remove from the pan immediately and let cool completely on a rack.

For a Loaf
3. Spoon batter into prepared loaf pan. Let stand for 30 minutes. Meanwhile, preheat oven to 350°F (180°C). Bake in preheated oven for 55 to 65 minutes, or until a cake tester inserted in the center comes out clean. Let cool in the pan on a rack for 10 minutes. Remove from the pan and let cool completely on a rack.

Poppy Seed Cheddar Muffins or Loaf

On a cold winter's day, serve these scrumptious golden morsels warm with a piping hot bowl of chili.

Tips

If muffins stick to the pan, let stand for 2 to 3 minutes, then try again to remove them.

For the amount of cheese to purchase, see the weight/volume equivalents in the Ingredient Glossary, page 174.

To heighten the cheese flavor, add a pinch of dry mustard.

If quinoa is not available, substitute an equal amount of brown rice flour.

Use two or three $5^1/_2$- by 3- by 2-inch (500 mL) pans and bake for 30 to 35 minutes.

12-cup muffin tin or 9- by 5-inch (2 L) loaf pan, lightly greased

1 cup	amaranth flour	250 mL
$1/_2$ cup	quinoa flour	125 mL
$1/_4$ cup	tapioca starch	50 mL
2 tbsp	granulated sugar	25 mL
$1^1/_2$ tsp	xanthan gum	7 mL
1 tbsp	GF baking powder	15 mL
$1/_2$ tsp	salt	2 mL
1 cup	shredded old Cheddar cheese	250 mL
2 tbsp	poppy seeds	25 mL
2	eggs	2
1 cup	milk	250 mL
2 tbsp	vegetable oil	25 mL
1 tsp	cider vinegar	5 mL

1. In a large bowl or plastic bag, combine amaranth flour, quinoa flour, tapioca starch, sugar, xanthan gum, baking powder, salt, Cheddar and poppy seeds. Mix well and set aside.
2. In a separate bowl, using an electric mixer, beat eggs, milk, oil and vinegar until combined. Add dry ingredients and mix just until combined.

For Muffins

3. Spoon batter evenly into each cup of prepared muffin tin. Let stand for 30 minutes. Meanwhile, preheat oven to 350°F (180°C). Bake in preheated oven for 18 to 20 minutes, or until firm to the touch. Remove from the pan immediately and let cool completely on a rack.

For a Loaf

3. Spoon batter into prepared loaf pan. Let stand for 30 minutes. Meanwhile, preheat oven to 350°F (180°C). Bake in preheated oven for 55 to 65 minutes, or until a cake tester inserted in the center comes out clean. Let cool in the pan on a rack for 10 minutes. Remove from the pan and let cool completely on a rack.

Pumpkin Muffins or Loaf

We love the colors of this quick bread. Bake as moist, spicy muffins or an easy-slicing, rich, dark loaf — or double the recipe and make both!

Tips

Be sure to buy pumpkin purée, not pumpkin pie filling, which is too sweet and contains too much moisture for this recipe.

Keep an eye on this one — it will become very dark as it bakes. You may need to tent the loaf with foil for the last 15 minutes. You will notice these are baked at a lower temperature than other muffins.

Toast pumpkin seeds for a nuttier flavor (see Techniques Glossary, page 181, under Sunflower seeds).

Vary the amount of cinnamon and nutmeg according to your tastes.

Substitute equal amounts of raisins and walnuts for the prunes and pumpkin seeds.

12-cup muffin tin or 9- by 5-inch (2 L) loaf pan, lightly greased

1/2 cup	sorghum flour	125 mL
1/2 cup	whole bean flour	125 mL
1/4 cup	tapioca starch	50 mL
1 1/2 tsp	xanthan gum	7 mL
2 tsp	GF baking powder	10 mL
1 tsp	baking soda	5 mL
1/2 tsp	salt	2 mL
1/2 cup	chopped prunes	125 mL
1/2 cup	pumpkin seeds	125 mL
1 tsp	ground cinnamon	5 mL
1/2 tsp	ground nutmeg	2 mL
2	eggs	2
1 cup	canned pumpkin purée	250 mL
1/3 cup	vegetable oil	75 mL
1 tsp	cider vinegar	5 mL
1/2 cup	liquid honey	125 mL

1. In a large bowl or plastic bag, combine sorghum flour, whole bean flour, tapioca starch, xanthan gum, baking powder, baking soda, salt, prunes, pumpkin seeds, cinnamon and nutmeg. Mix well and set aside.

2. In a separate bowl, using an electric mixer, beat eggs, pumpkin purée, oil and vinegar until combined. Add honey while mixing. Add dry ingredients and mix just until combined.

For Muffins

3. Spoon batter evenly into each cup of prepared muffin tin. Let stand for 30 minutes. Meanwhile, preheat oven to 325°F (160°C). Bake in preheated oven for 18 to 20 minutes, or until firm to the touch. Remove from the pan immediately and let cool completely on a rack.

For a Loaf

3. Spoon batter into prepared loaf pan. Let stand for 30 minutes. Meanwhile, preheat oven to 325°F (160°C). Bake in preheated oven for 55 to 65 minutes, or until a cake tester inserted in the center comes out clean. Let cool in the pan on a rack for 10 minutes. Remove from the pan and let cool completely on a rack.

Pineapple Banana Muffins or Loaf

Here's a delightfully moist, tender banana quick bread with bits of crushed pineapple throughout.

Tips

Be sure to include plenty of juice when spooning the crushed pineapple into the measuring cup.

If ground flaxseed is not available, purchase either golden or brown flaxseed and grind your own (see Techniques Glossary, page 180, for instructions). Whole flaxseed can be stored at room temperature for up to 1 year. Ground flaxseed can be stored in the refrigerator for up to 90 days, although for optimum freshness it is best to grind it as you need it.

Sometimes ground flaxseed is called flaxseed meal or flaxseed flour.

Substitute an equal amount of hempseed flour for the ground flaxseed.

12-cup muffin tin or 9 by 5-inch (2 L) loaf pan, lightly greased

1 cup	brown rice flour	250 mL
¾ cup	sorghum flour	175 mL
¼ cup	tapioca starch	50 mL
⅓ cup	ground flaxseed (see tip, at left)	75 mL
½ cup	granulated sugar	125 mL
1½ tsp	xanthan gum	7 mL
1 tbsp	GF baking powder	15 mL
½ tsp	salt	2 mL
1	egg	1
1	egg white	1
1 cup	crushed pineapple, including juice	250 mL
¾ cup	mashed banana	175 mL
2 tbsp	vegetable oil	25 mL
1 tsp	cider vinegar	5 mL

1. In a large bowl or plastic bag, combine brown rice flour, sorghum flour, tapioca starch, ground flaxseed, sugar, xanthan gum, baking powder and salt. Mix well and set aside.

2. In a separate bowl, using an electric mixer, beat egg, egg white, pineapple, banana, oil and vinegar until combined. Add dry ingredients and mix just until combined.

For Muffins

3. Spoon batter evenly into each cup of prepared muffin tin. Let stand for 30 minutes. Meanwhile, preheat oven to 350°F (180°C). Bake in preheated oven for 18 to 20 minutes, or until firm to the touch. Remove from the pan immediately and let cool completely on a rack.

For a Loaf

3. Spoon batter into prepared loaf pan. Let stand for 30 minutes. Meanwhile, preheat oven to 350°F (180°C). Bake in preheated oven for 55 to 65 minutes, or until a cake tester inserted in the center comes out clean. Let cool in the pan on a rack for 10 minutes. Remove from the pan and let cool completely on a rack.

Extra Baking Tips for Muffins, Loaves and More

- The batters should be the same consistency as wheat flour batters, but you can mix them more without producing tough products full of tunnels.
- Bake in muffin tins of a different size. Mini-muffins take 10 to 15 minutes to bake, while jumbo muffins bake in 20 to 40 minutes. Check jumbo muffins for doneness after 20 minutes, then again every 5 to 10 minutes. Keep in mind that the baking time will vary with the amount of batter in each muffin cup.
- Fill muffin tins to the top and loaf pans no more than three-quarters full. Let batter-filled pans stand for 30 minutes for a more tender product. It's worth the wait. We set a timer for 20 minutes, then preheat the oven so both are ready at the same time.
- If muffins stick to the lightly greased pan, let stand for a minute or two and try again. Loosen with a spatula or spoon if necessary.
- Muffins and biscuits can be reheated in the microwave, wrapped in a paper towel, for a few seconds on Medium (50%).

Make-Your-Own Quick Bread Mix

It's great to have this mix at the ready for those hectic days when your son reminds you it's his turn to provide a snack at school tomorrow or you remember you promised to bring the goodies for a Celiac Chapter meeting.

Tips

For added convenience, divide the mix into 5 portions, each about 2½ cups (625 mL), and store in resealable plastic bags in the freezer for up to 6 months. Label and date before freezing. We add the page number of the recipe to the label as a quick reference.

Soft brown sugar ensures even mixing.

Substitute any type of bean or pea flour for the garbanzo-fava bean flour.

3½ cups	sorghum flour	825 mL
2½ cups	amaranth flour	625 mL
2 cups	garbanzo-fava bean flour	500 mL
1 cup	quinoa flour	250 mL
1 cup	potato starch	250 mL
½ cup	tapioca starch	125 mL
½ cup	rice bran	125 mL
1¼ cups	packed brown sugar	300 mL
1 tbsp	xanthan gum	15 mL
¼ cup	GF baking powder	50 mL
2 tbsp	baking soda	25 mL
1 tbsp	salt	15 mL

1. In a very large bowl, combine the sorghum flour, amaranth flour, garbanzo-fava bean flour, quinoa flour, potato starch, tapioca starch, rice bran, brown sugar, xanthan gum, baking powder, baking soda and salt. Mix well.
2. Store dry mix in an airtight container in the freezer for up to 6 months. Allow to warm to room temperature and mix well before using.

Morning Glory Muffins or Loaf

With so many wonderfully fresh ingredients in this recipe, starting with our mix, you may want to double it and give the extra to neighbors.

Tips

Don't drain the pineapple; just spoon both juice and pulp into your measuring cup.

Substitute an equal amount of shredded zucchini for the carrots.

12-cup muffin tin or 9- by 5-inch (2 L) loaf pan, lightly greased

1/5 batch	Make-Your-Own Quick Bread Mix (see recipe, page 56)	1/5 batch
1/3 cup	unsweetened shredded coconut	75 mL
1/4 cup	raisins	50 mL
1 tbsp	grated lemon zest	15 mL
1 tsp	ground cinnamon	5 mL
2	eggs	2
1 cup	unsweetened applesauce	250 mL
2 tbsp	vegetable oil	25 mL
1 cup	shredded carrots	250 mL
1/2 cup	crushed pineapple, including juice	125 mL

1. In a large bowl or plastic bag, combine bread mix, coconut, raisins, lemon zest and cinnamon. Mix well and set aside.
2. In a separate bowl, using an electric mixer, beat eggs, applesauce and oil until combined. Stir in carrots and pineapple. Add dry ingredients and stir just until combined.

For Muffins
3. Spoon batter evenly into each cup of prepared muffin tin. Let stand for 30 minutes. Meanwhile, preheat oven to 350°F (180°C). Bake in preheated oven for 18 to 20 minutes, or until firm to the touch. Remove from the pan immediately and let cool completely on a rack.

For a Loaf
3. Spoon batter into prepared loaf pan. Let stand for 30 minutes. Meanwhile, preheat oven to 350°F (180°C). Bake in preheated oven for 55 to 65 minutes, or until a cake tester inserted in the center comes out clean. Let cool in the pan on a rack for 10 minutes. Remove from the pan and let cool completely on a rack.

Chocolate Orange Muffins or Loaf

Who can resist the combination of chocolate and orange? The buttermilk brings out the chocolate flavor without adding a lot of calories. The recipe is super-fast, as it begins with our mix.

Tips

The chocolate pieces will partially melt or remain whole depending on whether you use mini-chips, regular-size chips or chocolate chunks.

Top a thick slice of the loaf with a scoop of GF ice cream and Simple Hot Fudge Sauce (see recipe, page 157) for a last-minute fancy finale.

Instead of regular chocolate chips, try raspberry- or mint-flavored chocolate chips.

12-cup muffin tin or 9- by 5-inch (2 L) loaf pan, lightly greased

1/5 batch	Make-Your-Own Quick Bread Mix (see recipe, page 56)	1/5 batch
2/3 cup	semi-sweet chocolate chips	150 mL
1/4 cup	unsweetened cocoa powder, sifted	50 mL
2 tbsp	grated orange zest	25 mL
2	eggs	2
2/3 cup	buttermilk	150 mL
2/3 cup	freshly squeezed orange juice	150 mL
1/4 cup	vegetable oil	50 mL

1. In a large bowl or plastic bag, combine bread mix, chocolate chips, cocoa and orange zest. Mix well and set aside.

2. In a separate bowl, using an electric mixer, beat eggs, buttermilk, orange juice and oil until combined. Add dry ingredients and stir just until combined.

For Muffins

3. Spoon batter evenly into each cup of prepared muffin tin. Let stand for 30 minutes. Meanwhile, preheat oven to 350°F (180°C). Bake in preheated oven for 18 to 20 minutes, or until firm to the touch. Remove from the pan immediately and let cool completely on a rack.

For a Loaf

3. Spoon batter into prepared loaf pan. Let stand for 30 minutes. Meanwhile, preheat oven to 350°F (180°C). Bake in preheated oven for 55 to 65 minutes, or until a cake tester inserted in the center comes out clean. Let cool in the pan on a rack for 10 minutes. Remove from the pan and let cool completely on a rack.

Variation

To turn these muffins into sweeter cupcakes, add an extra 1 to 2 tbsp (15 to 25 mL) granulated sugar to the dry ingredients.

Apricot Date Muffins or Loaf

This tangy moist muffin that starts with our mix combines the complementary flavors of sweet dates, tart dried apricots and zesty orange. The perfect recipe for the time-pressured baker!

Tips

Use scissors to snip the dried apricots and dates. When the scissors become sticky, dip them in hot water.

We prefer to snip apricots into large pieces ourselves. The tiny slivers you sometimes purchase are too small to give a burst of flavor.

When purchasing chopped dates, check for wheat starch in the coating.

An equal amount of chopped pitted prunes can be substituted for either the apricots or the dates.

12-cup muffin tin or 9- by 5-inch (2 L) loaf pan, lightly greased

⅕ batch	Make-Your-Own Quick Bread Mix (see recipe, page 56)	⅕ batch
⅔ cup	chopped apricots	150 mL
⅔ cup	chopped pitted dates	150 mL
3 tbsp	grated orange zest	45 mL
1 tsp	ground nutmeg	5 mL
2	eggs	2
1¼ cups	plain yogurt	300 mL
2 tbsp	vegetable oil	25 mL

1. In a large bowl or plastic bag, combine bread mix, apricots, dates, orange zest and nutmeg. Mix well and set aside.
2. In a separate bowl, using an electric mixer, beat eggs, yogurt and oil until combined. Add dry ingredients and stir just until combined.

For Muffins

3. Spoon batter evenly into each cup of prepared muffin tin. Let stand for 30 minutes. Meanwhile, preheat oven to 350°F (180°C). Bake in preheated oven for 18 to 20 minutes, or until firm to the touch. Remove from the pan immediately and let cool completely on a rack.

For a Loaf

3. Spoon batter into prepared loaf pan. Let stand for 30 minutes. Meanwhile, preheat oven to 350°F (180°C). Bake in preheated oven for 55 to 65 minutes, or until a cake tester inserted in the center comes out clean. Let cool in the pan on a rack for 10 minutes. Remove from the pan and let cool completely on a rack.

Variation

Add ⅓ cup (75 mL) chopped dried apple with the apricots and dates.

Cheddar Bacon Muffins or Loaf

MAKES 12 MUFFINS OR 1 LOAF

Is there a cheese lover out there who doesn't enjoy Cheddar and bacon? Perfect with a salad for lunch.

Tips

Cook the bacon in the microwave for a crisper texture. Refer to your microwave manufacturer's "instructions for use" for power and time (it's usually about 1 minute per slice). Drain well on paper towels.

Substitute Swiss, GF Blue or GF Stilton cheese for the Cheddar.

12-cup muffin tin or 9- by 5-inch (2 L) loaf pan, lightly greased

6	slices GF bacon, cooked crisp and crumbled	6
1/5 batch	Make-Your-Own Quick Bread Mix (see recipe, page 56)	1/5 batch
3/4 cup	shredded old Cheddar cheese	175 mL
2/3 cup	snipped chives or green onion tops	150 mL
1/4 cup	freshly grated Parmesan cheese	50 mL
1/4 tsp	dry mustard	1 mL
2	eggs	2
1 cup	buttermilk	250 mL
2 tbsp	vegetable oil	25 mL

1. In a large bowl or plastic bag, combine bacon, bread mix, Cheddar, chives, Parmesan and mustard. Mix well and set aside.

2. In a separate bowl, using an electric mixer, beat eggs, buttermilk and oil until combined. Add dry ingredients and stir just until combined.

For Muffins

3. Spoon batter evenly into each cup of prepared muffin tin. Let stand for 30 minutes. Meanwhile, preheat oven to 350°F (180°C). Bake in preheated oven for 18 to 20 minutes, or until firm to the touch. Remove from the pan immediately and let cool completely on a rack.

For a Loaf

3. Spoon batter into prepared loaf pan. Let stand for 30 minutes. Meanwhile, preheat oven to 350°F (180°C). Bake in preheated oven for 50 to 60 minutes, or until a cake tester inserted in the center comes out clean. Let cool in the pan on a rack for 10 minutes. Remove from the pan and let cool completely on a rack.

Rhubarb Pistachio Muffins or Loaf

MAKES 12 MUFFINS OR 1 LOAF

Nothing heralds the arrival of spring more than a neighbor knocking on your door with an armful of rosy rhubarb. Use it to prepare this recipe, which starts with our mix. Little bits of tanginess dot this soft, slightly sweet treat — it's perfect for breakfast.

Tips

For easy slicing of the loaf, the rhubarb must be finely chopped.

Warm muffins or loaf slices in the microwave, wrapped in a paper towel, for 25 seconds on Medium (50%) power.

Substitute pecans or walnuts for the pistachios.

12-cup muffin tin or 9- by 5-inch (2 L) loaf pan, lightly greased

1/5 batch	Make-Your-Own Quick Bread Mix (see recipe, page 56)	1/5 batch
1/2 cup	chopped pistachios	125 mL
2 tbsp	granulated sugar	25 mL
2 tbsp	grated orange zest	25 mL
1 tsp	ground ginger	5 mL
2	eggs	2
2/3 cup	freshly squeezed orange juice	150 mL
1/4 cup	vegetable oil	50 mL
1 3/4 cups	finely chopped rhubarb	425 mL

1. In a large bowl or plastic bag, combine bread mix, pistachios, sugar, orange zest and ginger. Mix well and set aside.

2. In a separate bowl, using an electric mixer, beat eggs, orange juice and oil until combined. Stir in rhubarb. Add dry ingredients and stir just until combined.

For Muffins

3. Spoon batter evenly into each cup of prepared muffin tin. Let stand for 30 minutes. Meanwhile, preheat oven to 350°F (180°C). Bake in preheated oven for 18 to 20 minutes, or until firm to the touch. Remove from the pan immediately and let cool completely on a rack.

For a Loaf

3. Spoon batter into prepared loaf pan. Let stand for 30 minutes. Meanwhile, preheat oven to 350°F (180°C). Bake in preheated oven for 55 to 65 minutes, or until a cake tester inserted in the center comes out clean. Let cool in the pan on a rack for 10 minutes. Remove from the pan and let cool completely on a rack.

Currant Drop Biscuits with Honey Butter

MAKES 10 BISCUITS

Dried currants are a traditional ingredient in English tea biscuits. Here they're combined with a hint of orange. The honey butter makes a great accompaniment to these or any other biscuits.

Tips

Cold butter cuts more easily into dry ingredients than soft butter and produces flakier biscuits. For easier handling, cut the butter into 1-inch (2.5 cm) cubes before adding to dry mixture.

Honey butter can be stored, covered, in the refrigerator for up to 1 week. Bring to room temperature before serving.

For a change, try substituting an equal amount of golden raisins for the currants. Add raisins with the dry ingredients. They do not require soaking, so you can omit the water and skip Step 1.

Baking sheet, lightly greased

1 cup	boiling water	250 mL
1/3 cup	dried currants	75 mL
1 cup	amaranth flour	250 mL
1/2 cup	brown rice flour	125 mL
1/4 cup	granulated sugar	50 mL
1 1/2 tsp	xanthan gum	7 mL
2 tbsp	GF baking powder	25 mL
1/4 tsp	salt	1 mL
1 tbsp	grated orange zest	15 mL
1/4 cup	cold butter, cut into 1-inch (2.5 cm) cubes (see tip, at left)	50 mL
3/4 cup	milk	175 mL

HONEY BUTTER

1/2 cup	butter, softened	125 mL
1/4 cup	creamed honey	50 mL
2 tsp	grated orange zest	10 mL

1. In a small bowl, pour boiling water over currants. Let stand for 5 minutes. Drain currants well and pat dry on paper towels. Set aside.

2. In a large bowl, combine amaranth flour, brown rice flour, sugar, xanthan gum, baking powder, salt and orange zest. Using a pastry blender or two knives, cut in butter until mixture resembles coarse crumbs. Stir in currants. Add milk all at once, stirring with a fork to make a soft, slightly sticky dough. Drop by heaping spoonfuls onto prepared baking sheet. Let stand for 30 minutes. Meanwhile, preheat oven to 425°F (220°C).

3. Bake in preheated oven for 10 to 13 minutes, or until tops are golden. Remove biscuits immediately to a cooling rack.

4. *Prepare the honey butter:* In a small bowl, cream together butter, honey and orange zest. Serve with warm biscuits.

Triple Cheese Scones

You'll be easily tempted to go back for seconds of these cheesy biscuits. Serve hot with a steaming bowl of soup on a cold winter's day.

Tips

While the oven is preheating, you have plenty of time to prepare these scones for baking.

For quick and easy serving, cut into wedges with a pizza cutter.

Warm in the microwave, wrapped in a paper towel, for 25 seconds on Medium (50%) power. Scones become rubbery when overheated.

Add ¼ cup (50 mL) snipped fresh parsley and 1½ tsp (7 mL) snipped fresh dill, rosemary, marjoram or savory to the dry ingredients to make a cheese-herb scone.

Try adding 6 slices of cooked crisp crumbled bacon to the dry ingredients.

9-inch (2.5 L) round baking pan, ungreased

¾ cup	almond flour	175 mL
¾ cup	brown rice flour	175 mL
3 tbsp	granulated sugar	45 mL
1 tsp	xanthan gum	5 mL
1 tbsp	GF baking powder	15 mL
1 tsp	baking soda	5 mL
¼ tsp	salt	1 mL
3 tbsp	freshly grated Parmesan cheese	45 mL
Pinch	dry mustard	Pinch
¼ cup	shortening or butter	50 mL
¾ cup	shredded Swiss cheese	175 mL
¼ cup	crumbled GF blue cheese	50 mL
¾ cup	plain yogurt	175 mL

Traditional Method

1. In a large bowl, combine almond flour, brown rice flour, sugar, xanthan gum, baking powder, baking soda, salt, Parmesan and dry mustard. Using a pastry blender or two knives, cut in shortening until mixture resembles coarse crumbs. Stir in Swiss and blue cheese. Add yogurt all at once, stirring with a fork to make a soft, sticky dough.

Food Processor Method

1. In a food processor fitted with a metal blade, pulse almond flour, brown rice flour, sugar, xanthan gum, baking powder, baking soda, salt, Parmesan and dry mustard. Add shortening, Swiss and blue cheese and pulse until mixture resembles small peas, about 5 to 10 seconds. Add yogurt and pulse 3 or 4 times, until dough just holds together. Do not over-process.

For Both Methods

2. Spoon dough into pan, leaving top rough. Let stand for 30 minutes. Meanwhile, preheat oven to 425°F (220°C). Bake in preheated oven for 20 to 25 minutes, or until top is golden. Remove immediately to a cooling rack. Cut into 8 wedges and serve hot.

Southern Cornbread

Here's a new twist on an old favorite — traditional cornbread nutritionally enhanced with amaranth flour, an excellent source of high-quality protein. Serve hot from the oven with soup, a salad or a casserole.

Tips
Amaranth flour provides iron, calcium and fiber as well as protein.

An equal amount of light or regular pancake syrup or liquid honey can be substituted for the maple syrup.

9-inch (2.5 L) square baking pan, lightly greased

1 cup	amaranth flour	250 mL
1¼ cups	cornmeal	300 mL
1½ tsp	xanthan gum	7 mL
2 tsp	GF baking powder	10 mL
1 tsp	baking soda	5 mL
½ tsp	salt	2 mL
2	eggs	2
1 cup	buttermilk	250 mL
⅓ cup	vegetable oil	75 mL
⅓ cup	pure maple syrup	75 mL

1. In a large bowl or plastic bag, combine amaranth flour, cornmeal, xanthan gum, baking powder, baking soda and salt. Mix well and set aside.

2. In a separate bowl, using an electric mixer, beat eggs, buttermilk, oil and maple syrup until combined. Add dry ingredients and mix just until combined. Spoon into prepared pan. Let stand for 30 minutes. Meanwhile, preheat oven to 350°F (180°C).

4. Bake in preheated oven for 25 to 30 minutes, or until a cake tester inserted in the center comes out clean. Serve hot.

Variation
Jazz up this cornbread with 3 slices of cooked crisp crumbled bacon and hot pepper flakes to taste.

Mediterranean Focaccia (page 82)

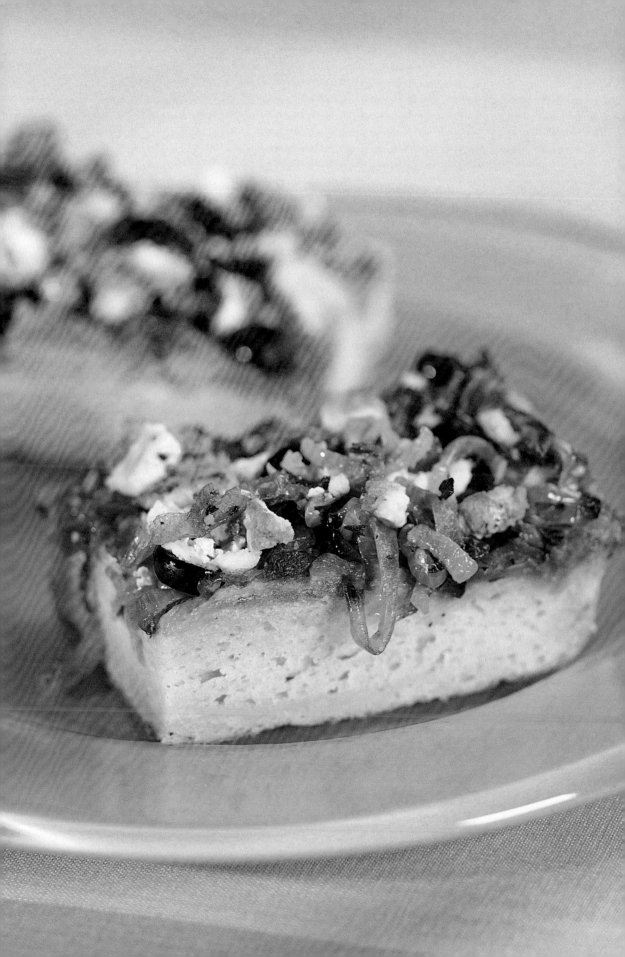

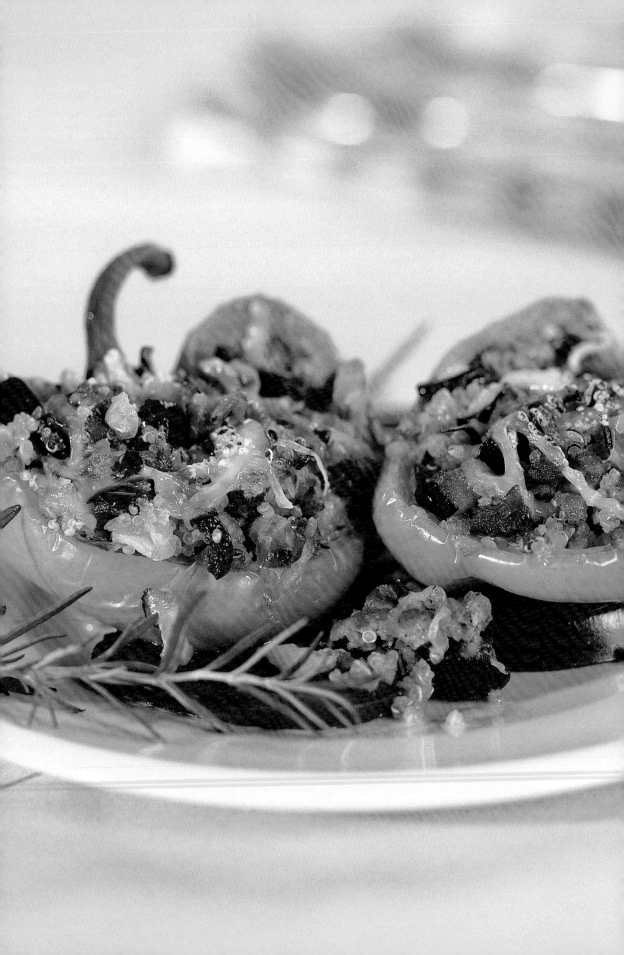

Bread Machine & Mixer-Method Yeast Breads

Tired of plain white bread? Try these!

Quinoa-Stuffed Peppers (page 104)

A Page from Deanna's Diary

IT'S REALLY HARD BEING A KID WITH CELIAC DISEASE. It's hard enough just feeling different, but you also have to learn to cope seeing all of your friends eating pizza and other foods you can't have. You know sometimes you are not being invited to parties because you are different. Some parents just don't want to have to deal with it, maybe they just don't want to ask questions, or maybe they are afraid of making me sick. On the other hand, getting invited to something, you or your parent has to figure out what you are going to eat. It usually works best if you offer to bring something for yourself, like a frozen pizza or a cupcake. If you know the family really well, they might want to take on the challenge of trying to make something that you can eat — keep your requests simple and it will work.

If you like to go out for dinner with your friends, then you should probably go to a restaurant that you are familiar with and know ahead of time what you can order. School lunches can be difficult, but try salads with cubes of cheese, a cooked and cooled grilled cheese sandwich, sliced cheese and rice crackers or corn chips with salsa.

If your school has a cafeteria, you need to check if there is anything you can have, so don't be afraid to ask questions. You may even be able to have the french fries if they are cooked in a separate fryer. If you can keep some snacks at school, either yourself or with your teacher, you can be part of food celebrations and contests too.

Make sure you tell your friends what you can and can't have so that they know and will not try to interfere with your food. It's hard not getting as much food or celebration time with your friends, but it's worth it to be healthy and feel good. You're not alone — there are lots of kids with celiac disease just like you.

— *Deanna Jennett, Kingston, Ontario, a young lady living with celiac disease*

Baking Bread Machine Yeast Breads

- The recipes were developed for 1.5 lb (750 g) and 2 lb (1 kg) bread machines with a Rapid Two-Hour Basic Cycle, a Dough then a Bake Cycle, or a programmable mode. A 58-Minute Rapid Cycle or 70-Minute Rapid Cycle are not long enough to rise and bake the loaves successfully.
- When using the Dough then Bake Cycle, keep an eye on the machine to see whether it knocks down the dough just before the Dough Cycle ends. If it does, stop the cycle 5 minutes before the end. (Set a separate kitchen timer to remind you.) The dough is risen and ready to bake. Just press the Bake Cycle. There's no need to handle the dough.
- Instant or bread machine yeast becomes inactive at high temperatures, and bread won't rise. To be on the safe side, test the temperature of the water with an instant-read thermometer before adding it to the baking pan. It should be between 120°F (50°C) and 130°F (55°C).
- If your bread machine has a preheat, keep the top down until it starts so the heat doesn't escape. As soon as the liquids begin to mix, add the dry ingredients, scraping the sides and bottom of the baking pan with a rubber spatula. Watch that the spatula does not get caught under the blade. Quickly close the top.
- The dough should be the consistency of a thick batter. You can see the mixing pattern of the blade in the batter.
- Removing the blade as soon as the long knead is done prevents over-kneading and a collapsed loaf. Set a kitchen timer so you won't miss it. The dough will be sticky, so wet your fingers and a spatula. Smooth the top quickly once the paddle is removed.
- At the end of the cycle, before turning off the bread machine, take the temperature of the loaf using an instant-read thermometer. It should read 200°F (100°C). If it hasn't reached the recommended temperature, leave the loaf in the machine for 10 to 15 minutes on the Keep Warm Cycle.

Baking Mixer-Method Yeast Breads

- Select a heavy-duty mixer with a paddle attachment for the best mixing of ingredients.
- Add the dry ingredients slowly to the liquids as the machine is mixing. Stop the machine and scrape the bottom and sides of the bowl.
- With the mixer set to medium speed, beat the dough for 4 minutes. Set a kitchen timer. You will be surprised how long 4 minutes seems when you are waiting.
- Fill the lightly greased pan only two-thirds full, then set, uncovered, in a warm, draft-free place until the dough reaches the top of the pan. This usually takes 60 to 75 minutes. Do not let over-rise, or the loaf could collapse during baking.
- After baking, take the temperature of the loaf using an instant-read thermometer. It should read 200°F (100°C). If it doesn't, continue baking until it does. Remove from pan and place loaf on a rack immediately to prevent a soggy loaf.

Cinnamon Raisin Bread
(Bread Machine Method)

MAKES 1 LOAF

Enjoy a toasted slice or two of this deep golden loaf for breakfast — it's the perfect snack when served with a cup of hot cocoa.

Tips

To ensure success, see page 67 for extra information on baking yeast bread in a bread machine.

Water at 130°F (55°C) will feel hot to the touch.

Thoroughly mix the dry ingredients before adding them to the liquids — they are powder-fine and can clump together.

Substitute other dried fruits for the raisins — try cranberries, currants, apricots or a mixture.

1¾ cups	rice flour	425 mL
½ cup	potato starch	125 mL
¼ cup	tapioca starch	50 mL
½ cup	granulated sugar	125 mL
¼ cup	nonfat (skim) milk powder	50 mL
1 tbsp	xanthan gum	15 mL
1 tbsp	bread machine or instant yeast	15 mL
1¼ tsp	salt	6 mL
1 tbsp	ground cinnamon	15 mL
1 cup	water, warmed to 130°F (55°C)	250 mL
2 tbsp	vegetable oil	25 mL
2 tsp	cider vinegar	10 mL
2	eggs	2
2	egg whites	2
1½ cups	raisins	375 mL

1. In a large bowl or plastic bag, combine rice flour, potato starch, tapioca starch, sugar, milk powder, xanthan gum, yeast, salt and cinnamon. Mix well and set aside.

2. Pour water, oil and vinegar into the bread machine baking pan. Add eggs and egg whites.

3. Select the **Rapid Two-Hour Basic Cycle**. Allow the liquids to mix until combined. As the bread machine is mixing, gradually add the dry ingredients, scraping bottom and sides of pan with a rubber spatula. Incorporate all the dry ingredients within 1 to 2 minutes. Add raisins.

4. When the mixing and kneading are complete, remove the kneading blade, leaving the bread pan in the bread machine. Quickly smooth the top of the loaf. Allow the bread machine to complete the cycle. Remove loaf from the pan immediately and let cool completely on a rack.

Cinnamon Raisin Bread
(Mixer Method)

Enjoy a toasted slice or two of this deep golden loaf for breakfast — it's the perfect snack when served with a cup of hot cocoa.

Tips

To ensure success, see page 67 for extra information on baking yeast bread using the mixer method.

Thoroughly mix the dry ingredients before adding them to the liquids — they are powder-fine and can clump together.

Substitute other dried fruits for the raisins — try cranberries, currants, apricots or a mixture.

9- by 5-inch (2 L) loaf pan, lightly greased

1½ cups	rice flour	375 mL
⅓ cup	potato starch	75 mL
¼ cup	tapioca starch	50 mL
¼ cup	nonfat (skim) milk powder	50 mL
⅓ cup	granulated sugar	75 mL
1 tbsp	xanthan gum	15 mL
1 tbsp	bread machine or instant yeast	15 mL
1¼ tsp	salt	6 mL
2 tsp	cinnamon	10 mL
2	eggs	2
1	egg white	1
1 cup	water	250 mL
2 tbsp	vegetable oil	25 mL
1 tsp	cider vinegar	5 mL
1¼ cups	raisins	300 mL

1. In a large bowl or plastic bag, combine rice flour, potato starch, tapioca starch, milk powder, sugar, xanthan gum, yeast, salt and cinnamon. Mix well and set aside.

2. In a separate bowl, using a heavy-duty electric mixer with paddle attachment, combine eggs, egg white, water, oil and vinegar until well blended. With the mixer on its lowest speed, slowly add the dry ingredients until combined. Stop the machine and scrape the bottom and sides of the bowl with a rubber spatula. With the mixer on medium speed, beat for 4 minutes. Stir in raisins.

3. Spoon into prepared pan. Let rise, uncovered, in a warm, draft-free place for 75 to 90 minutes, or until dough has risen to the top of the pan. Meanwhile, preheat oven to 350°F (180°C).

4. Bake for 35 to 45 minutes, or until loaf sounds hollow when tapped on the bottom. Remove from the pan immediately and let cool completely on a rack.

Italian Herb Bread
(Bread Machine Method)

The fragrant aroma of this loaf makes waiting for it to bake extremely difficult. Serve this zesty herb bread with any course — soup, salad or entrée.

Tips

To ensure success, see page 67 for extra information on baking yeast bread in a bread machine.

Water at 130°F (55°C) will feel hot to the touch.

This is an excellent loaf for making croutons and bread crumbs (see Techniques Glossary, page 179).

Substitute triple the amount of snipped fresh herbs for the dried. See Techniques Glossary, page 180, for information about working with fresh herbs.

1½ cups	sorghum flour	375 mL
¾ cup	whole bean flour	175 mL
½ cup	potato starch	125 mL
¼ cup	tapioca starch	50 mL
⅓ cup	granulated sugar	75 mL
1 tbsp	xanthan gum	15 mL
2 tsp	bread machine or instant yeast	10 mL
1½ tsp	salt	7 mL
¼ cup	snipped fresh parsley	50 mL
1 tbsp	ground dried marjoram	15 mL
1 tbsp	ground dried thyme	15 mL
1¼ cups	water, warmed to 130°F (55°C)	300 mL
⅓ cup	vegetable oil	75 mL
1 tsp	cider vinegar	5 mL
2	eggs	2

1. In a large bowl or plastic bag, combine sorghum flour, whole bean flour, potato starch, tapioca starch, sugar, xanthan gum, yeast, salt, parsley, marjoram and thyme. Mix well and set aside.

2. Pour water, oil and vinegar into the bread machine baking pan. Add eggs.

3. Select the **Rapid Two-Hour Basic Cycle**. Allow the liquids to mix until combined. As the bread machine is mixing, gradually add the dry ingredients, scraping bottom and sides of pan with a rubber spatula. Try to incorporate all the dry ingredients within 1 to 2 minutes.

4. When the mixing and kneading are complete, remove the kneading blade, leaving the bread pan in the bread machine. Quickly smooth the top of the loaf. Allow the bread machine to complete the cycle. Remove loaf from the pan immediately and let cool completely on a rack.

Italian Herb Bread
(Mixer Method)

MAKES 1 LOAF

The fragrant aroma of this loaf makes waiting for it to bake extremely difficult. Serve this zesty herb bread with any course — soup, salad or entrée.

Tips

To ensure success, see page 67 for extra information on baking yeast bread using the mixer method.

This is an excellent loaf for making croutons and bread crumbs (see Techniques Glossary, page 179).

Substitute triple the amount of snipped fresh herbs for the dried. See Techniques Glossary, page 180, for information about working with fresh herbs.

9- by 5-inch (2 L) loaf pan, lightly greased

1¼ cups	sorghum flour	300 mL
½ cup	whole bean flour	125 mL
⅓ cup	potato starch	75 mL
⅓ cup	tapioca starch	75 mL
¼ cup	granulated sugar	50 mL
2½ tsp	xanthan gum	12 mL
2 tsp	bread machine or instant yeast	10 mL
1¼ tsp	salt	7 mL
¼ cup	snipped fresh parsley	50 mL
2 tsp	ground dried marjoram	10 mL
2 tsp	ground dried thyme	10 mL
2	eggs	2
1¼ cups	water	300 mL
¼ cup	vegetable oil	50 mL
1 tsp	cider vinegar	5 mL

1. In a large bowl or plastic bag, combine sorghum flour, whole bean flour, potato starch, tapioca starch, sugar, xanthan gum, yeast, salt, parsley, marjoram and thyme. Mix well and set aside.

2. In a separate bowl, using a heavy-duty electric mixer with paddle attachment, combine eggs, water, oil and vinegar until well blended. With the mixer on its lowest speed, slowly add the dry ingredients until combined. Stop the machine and scrape the bottom and sides of the bowl with a rubber spatula. With the mixer on medium speed, beat for 4 minutes.

3. Spoon into prepared pan. Let rise, uncovered, in a warm, draft-free place for 60 to 75 minutes, or until dough has risen to the top of the pan. Meanwhile, preheat oven to 350°F (180°C).

4. Bake for 35 to 45 minutes, or until loaf sounds hollow when tapped on the bottom. Remove from the pan immediately and let cool completely on a rack.

Whole Grain Amaranth Bread
(Bread Machine Method)

This soft-textured, creamy, honey-colored bread is so delicious you won't even suspect how nutritious it is.

Tips

To ensure success, see page 67 for extra information on baking yeast bread in a bread machine.

Water at 130°F (55°C) will feel hot to the touch.

Substitute ¼ cup (50 mL) liquid egg whites for the 2 egg whites.

Store amaranth grain in an airtight container in the refrigerator for up to 6 months.

Amaranth is high in fiber, iron and calcium and lower in sodium than most grains.

1¼ cups	brown rice flour	300 mL
¾ cup	amaranth flour	175 mL
½ cup	potato starch	125 mL
⅓ cup	amaranth grain	75 mL
1 tbsp	xanthan gum	15 mL
2 tsp	bread machine or instant yeast	10 mL
1½ tsp	salt	7 mL
2 tbsp	grated orange zest	25 mL
1 cup	water, warmed to 130°F (55°C)	250 mL
¼ cup	vegetable oil	50 mL
¼ cup	liquid honey	50 mL
2 tsp	cider vinegar	10 mL
2	eggs	2
2	egg whites	2

1. In a large bowl or plastic bag, combine brown rice flour, amaranth flour, potato starch, amaranth grain, xanthan gum, yeast, salt and orange zest. Mix well and set aside.

2. Pour water, oil, honey and vinegar into the bread machine baking pan. Add eggs and egg whites.

3. Select the **Rapid Two-Hour Basic Cycle**. Allow the liquids to mix until combined. As the bread machine is mixing, gradually add the dry ingredients, scraping bottom and sides of pan with a rubber spatula. Try to incorporate all the dry ingredients within 1 to 2 minutes.

4. When the mixing and kneading are complete, remove the kneading blade, leaving the bread pan in the bread machine. Quickly smooth the top of the loaf. Allow the bread machine to complete the cycle. Remove loaf from the pan immediately and let cool completely on a rack.

Whole Grain Amaranth Bread
(Mixer Method)

This soft-textured, creamy, honey-colored bread is so delicious you won't even suspect how nutritious it is.

Tips

To ensure success, see page 67 for extra information on baking yeast bread using the mixer method.

Substitute ¼ cup (50 mL) liquid egg whites for the 2 egg whites.

Store amaranth grain in an airtight container in the refrigerator for up to 6 months.

Amaranth is high in fiber, iron and calcium and lower in sodium than most grains.

9- by 5-inch (2 L) loaf pan, lightly greased

1 cup	brown rice flour	250 mL
⅔ cup	amaranth flour	150 mL
½ cup	potato starch	125 mL
¼ cup	amaranth grain	50 mL
1 tbsp	xanthan gum	15 mL
2 tsp	bread machine or instant yeast	10 mL
1¼ tsp	salt	6 mL
2 tbsp	grated orange zest	25 mL
2	eggs	2
2	egg whites	2
¾ cup	water	175 mL
3 tbsp	vegetable oil	45 mL
3 tbsp	liquid honey	45 mL
2 tsp	cider vinegar	10 mL

1. In a large bowl or plastic bag, combine brown rice flour, amaranth flour, potato starch, amaranth grain, xanthan gum, yeast, salt and orange zest. Mix well and set aside.

2. In a separate bowl, using a heavy-duty electric mixer with paddle attachment, combine eggs, egg whites, water, oil, honey and vinegar until well blended. With the mixer on its lowest speed, slowly add the dry ingredients until combined. Stop the machine and scrape the bottom and sides of the bowl with a rubber spatula. With the mixer on medium speed, beat for 4 minutes.

3. Spoon into prepared pan. Let rise, uncovered, in a warm, draft-free place for 70 to 80 minutes, or until dough has risen to the top of the pan. Meanwhile, preheat oven to 350°F (180°C).

4. Bake for 35 to 45 minutes, or until loaf sounds hollow when tapped on the bottom. Remove from the pan immediately and let cool completely on a rack.

Seedy Brown Bread
(Bread Machine Method)

A sandwich bread with a rich color and added crunch — what a treat!

Tips

To ensure success, see page 67 for extra information on baking yeast bread in a bread machine.

Water at 130°F (55°C) will feel hot to the touch.

You can purchase buttermilk powder in bulk stores and health food stores.

For a nuttier flavor, toast the seeds (see Techniques Glossary, page 181).

To crack flaxseeds, pulse in a coffee grinder to desired texture.

For a milder-flavored bread, substitute packed brown sugar for the molasses.

Rice bran can be replaced by an equal amount of brown rice flour.

See page 75 for more tips.

1 cup	sorghum flour	250 mL
2/3 cup	whole bean flour	150 mL
1/3 cup	tapioca starch	75 mL
1/3 cup	rice bran	75 mL
1/3 cup	buttermilk powder	75 mL
1 tbsp	xanthan gum	15 mL
1 tbsp	bread machine or instant yeast	15 mL
1 1/4 tsp	salt	6 mL
1/3 cup	pumpkin seeds	75 mL
1/3 cup	raw unsalted sunflower seeds	75 mL
1/4 cup	sesame seeds	50 mL
1 cup	water, warmed to 130°F (55°C)	250 mL
2 tbsp	vegetable oil	25 mL
2 tbsp	liquid honey	25 mL
2 tbsp	fancy molasses	25 mL
1 tsp	cider vinegar	5 mL
3	eggs	3

1. In a large bowl or plastic bag, combine sorghum flour, whole bean flour, tapioca starch, rice bran, buttermilk powder, xanthan gum, yeast, salt and pumpkin, sunflower and sesame seeds. Mix well and set aside.

2. Pour water, oil, honey, molasses and vinegar into the bread machine baking pan. Add eggs.

3. Select the **Rapid Two-Hour Basic Cycle**. Allow the liquids to mix until combined. As the bread machine is mixing, gradually add the dry ingredients, scraping bottom and sides of pan with a rubber spatula. Try to incorporate all the dry ingredients within 1 to 2 minutes.

4. When the mixing and kneading are complete, remove the kneading blade, leaving the bread pan in the bread machine. Quickly smooth the top of the loaf. Allow the bread machine to complete the cycle. Remove loaf from the pan immediately and let cool completely on a rack.

Seedy Brown Bread
(Mixer Method)

MAKES 1 LOAF

A sandwich bread with a rich color and added crunch — what a treat!

Tips

To ensure success, see page 67 for extra information on baking yeast bread using the mixer method.

Store buttermilk powder in an airtight container to prevent lumping.

Tent the loaf with foil partway through the baking time to prevent the top crust from becoming too dark.

Vary the seeds — choose either flax, hemp or poppy to substitute for the sesame.

Substitute raw hemp powder or flaxseed meal for the rice bran.

See page 74 for more tips.

9- by 5-inch (2 L) loaf pan, lightly greased

1 cup	sorghum flour	250 mL
1/2 cup	whole bean flour	125 mL
1/3 cup	tapioca starch	75 mL
1/4 cup	rice bran	50 mL
1/3 cup	buttermilk powder	75 mL
1 tbsp	xanthan gum	15 mL
1 tbsp	bread machine or instant yeast	15 mL
1 1/4 tsp	salt	6 mL
1/4 cup	pumpkin seeds	50 mL
1/4 cup	raw unsalted sunflower seeds	50 mL
1/4 cup	sesame seeds	50 mL
2	eggs	2
1 cup	water	250 mL
2 tbsp	vegetable oil	25 mL
2 tbsp	liquid honey	25 mL
1 tbsp	fancy molasses	15 mL
1 tsp	cider vinegar	5 mL

1. In a large bowl or plastic bag, combine sorghum flour, whole bean flour, tapioca starch, rice bran, buttermilk powder, xanthan gum, yeast, salt and pumpkin, sunflower and sesame seeds. Mix well and set aside.

2. In a separate bowl, using a heavy-duty electric mixer with paddle attachment, combine eggs, water, oil, honey, molasses and vinegar until well blended. With the mixer on its lowest speed, slowly add the dry ingredients until combined. Stop the machine and scrape the bottom and sides of the bowl with a rubber spatula. With the mixer on medium speed, beat for 4 minutes.

3. Spoon into prepared pan. Let rise, uncovered, in a warm, draft-free place for 70 to 80 minutes, or until dough has risen to the top of the pan. Meanwhile, preheat oven to 350°F (180°C).

4. Bake for 35 to 45 minutes, or until loaf sounds hollow when tapped on the bottom. Remove from the pan immediately and let cool completely on a rack.

Daffodil Loaf
(Bread Machine Method)

Bring a little bit of springtime to your table! Enjoy this bread's light, cake-like texture, with its refreshing aroma and flavor of orange. Serve for a mid-morning coffee break.

Tips

To ensure success, see page 67 for extra information on baking yeast bread in a bread machine.

Water at 130°F (55°C) will feel hot to the touch.

For thin, even slices, use an electric knife for this and all breads.

Substitute lime or three-fruit marmalade for the orange marmalade.

1½ cups	brown rice flour	375 mL
¾ cup	quinoa flour	175 mL
½ cup	arrowroot starch	125 mL
¼ cup	tapioca starch	50 mL
1 tbsp	xanthan gum	15 mL
1 tbsp	bread machine or instant yeast	15 mL
1¼ tsp	salt	6 mL
1 cup	water, warmed to 130°F (55°C)	250 mL
¼ cup	vegetable oil	50 mL
3 tbsp	frozen orange juice concentrate, thawed	45 mL
2	eggs	2
½ cup	Orange Marmalade (see recipe, page 90)	125 mL

1. In a large bowl or plastic bag, combine brown rice flour, quinoa flour, arrowroot starch, tapioca starch, xanthan gum, yeast and salt. Mix well and set aside.
2. Pour water, oil and orange juice concentrate into the bread machine baking pan. Add eggs and marmalade.
3. Select the **Rapid Two-Hour Basic Cycle**. Allow the liquids to mix until combined. As the bread machine is mixing, gradually add the dry ingredients, scraping bottom and sides of pan with a rubber spatula. Try to incorporate all the dry ingredients within 1 to 2 minutes.
4. When the mixing and kneading are complete, remove the kneading blade, leaving the bread pan in the bread machine. Quickly smooth the top of the loaf. Allow the bread machine to complete the cycle. Remove loaf from the pan immediately and let cool completely on a rack.

Daffodil Loaf
(Mixer Method)

Bring a little bit of springtime to your table! Enjoy this bread's light, cake-like texture, with its refreshing aroma and flavor of orange. Serve for a mid-morning coffee break.

Tips

To ensure success, see page 67 for extra information on baking yeast bread using the mixer method.

For thin, even slices, use an electric knife for this and all breads.

Substitute lime or three-fruit marmalade for the orange marmalade.

9- by 5-inch (2 L) loaf pan, lightly greased

1 1/4 cups	brown rice flour	300 mL
1/3 cup	quinoa flour	75 mL
1/3 cup	arrowroot starch	75 mL
1/4 cup	tapioca starch	50 mL
1 tbsp	xanthan gum	15 mL
1 tbsp	bread machine or instant yeast	15 mL
1 1/4 tsp	salt	6 mL
2	eggs	2
3/4 cup	water	175 mL
1/3 cup	Orange Marmalade (see recipe, page 90)	75 mL
1/4 cup	vegetable oil	50 mL
3 tbsp	frozen orange juice concentrate, thawed	45 mL

1. In a large bowl or plastic bag, combine brown rice flour, quinoa flour, arrowroot starch, tapioca starch, xanthan gum, yeast and salt. Mix well and set aside.

2. In a separate bowl, using a heavy-duty electric mixer with paddle attachment, combine eggs, water, marmalade, oil and orange juice concentrate until well blended. With the mixer on its lowest speed, slowly add the dry ingredients until combined. Stop the machine and scrape the bottom and sides of the bowl with a rubber spatula. With the mixer on medium speed, beat for 4 minutes.

3. Spoon into prepared pan. Let rise, uncovered, in a warm, draft-free place for 60 to 75 minutes, or until dough has risen to the top of the pan. Meanwhile, preheat oven to 350°F (180°C).

4. Bake for 35 to 45 minutes, or until loaf sounds hollow when tapped on the bottom. Remove from the pan immediately and let cool completely on a rack.

Henk's Flax Bread
(Bread Machine Method)

MAKES 1 LOAF

Henk Rietveld of Huntsville, Ontario, a recipe tester and member of the focus group for this book, suggested using the flax flour in this loaf.

Tips

To ensure success, see page 67 for extra information on baking yeast bread in a bread machine.

Water at 130°F (55°C) will feel hot to the touch.

We tried this bread with sprouted flax powder, flax meal, ground flaxseed and flax flour, and there were really no differences.

This bread is delicious thinly sliced and toasted.

Substitute raw hemp powder and hemp hearts® for flax, both flour and seeds.

Substitute an equal amount of packed brown sugar for the honey.

1 1/3 cups	brown rice flour	325 mL
1/3 cup	flax flour	75 mL
2/3 cup	potato starch	150 mL
1/3 cup	cornstarch	75 mL
1/3 cup	cracked flaxseed (see Techniques Glossary, page 180)	75 mL
1/3 cup	nonfat (skim) milk powder	75 mL
2 1/2 tsp	xanthan gum	12 mL
2 1/4 tsp	bread machine or instant yeast	11 mL
1 1/2 tsp	salt	7 mL
1 1/4 cups	water, warmed to 130°F (55°C)	300 mL
1/4 cup	vegetable oil	50 mL
1/4 cup	liquid honey	50 mL
2 tsp	cider vinegar	10 mL
2	eggs	2
2	egg whites	2

1. In a large bowl or plastic bag, combine rice flour, flax flour, potato starch, cornstarch, flaxseed, milk powder, xanthan gum, yeast and salt. Mix well and set aside.

2. Pour water, oil, honey and vinegar into the bread machine baking pan. Add eggs and egg whites.

3. Select the **Rapid Two-Hour Basic Cycle**. Allow the liquids to mix until combined. As the bread machine is mixing, gradually add the dry ingredients, scraping bottom and sides of pan with a rubber spatula. Try to incorporate all the dry ingredients within 1 to 2 minutes.

4. When the mixing and kneading are complete, remove the kneading blade, leaving the bread pan in the bread machine. Quickly smooth the top of the loaf. Allow the bread machine to complete the cycle. Remove loaf from the pan immediately and let cool completely on a rack.

Henk's Flax Bread
(Mixer Method)

MAKES 1 LOAF

Henk Rietveld of Huntsville, Ontario, a recipe tester and member of the focus group for this book, suggested using the flax flour in this loaf.

Tips

To ensure success, see page 67 for extra information on baking yeast bread using the mixer method.

We tried this bread with sprouted flax powder, flax meal, ground flaxseed and flax flour, and there were really no differences.

This bread is delicious thinly sliced and toasted.

Substitute raw hemp powder and hemp hearts® for flax, both flour and seeds.

Substitute an equal amount of packed brown sugar for the honey.

9- by 5-inch (2 L) loaf pan, lightly greased

1¼ cups	brown rice flour	300 mL
¼ cup	flax flour	50 mL
½ cup	potato starch	125 mL
¼ cup	cornstarch	50 mL
¼ cup	cracked flaxseed (see Techniques Glossary, page 180)	50 mL
¼ cup	nonfat (skim) milk powder	50 mL
2½ tsp	xanthan gum	12 mL
2 tsp	bread machine or instant yeast	10 mL
1¼ tsp	salt	6 mL
2	eggs	2
2	egg whites	2
1 cup	water	250 mL
2 tbsp	vegetable oil	25 mL
2 tbsp	liquid honey	25 mL
2 tsp	cider vinegar	10 mL

1. In a large bowl or plastic bag, combine rice flour, flax flour, potato starch, cornstarch, flaxseed, milk powder, xanthan gum, yeast and salt. Mix well and set aside.

2. In a separate bowl, using a heavy-duty electric mixer with paddle attachment, combine eggs, egg whites, water, oil, honey and vinegar until well blended. With the mixer on its lowest speed, slowly add the dry ingredients until combined. Stop the machine and scrape the bottom and sides of the bowl with a rubber spatula. With the mixer on medium speed, beat for 4 minutes.

3. Spoon into prepared pan. Let rise, uncovered, in a warm, draft-free place for 60 to 75 minutes, or until dough has risen to the top of the pan. Meanwhile, preheat oven to 350°F (180°C).

4. Bake for 35 to 45 minutes, or until loaf sounds hollow when tapped on the bottom. Remove from the pan immediately and let cool completely on a rack.

Focaccia

MAKES 2 FOCACCIA

Plan to serve this chewy flatbread hot from the oven along with soup or salad lunches, or cut into small pieces and serve as hors d'oeuvres.

Tips

To ensure success, see page 67 for extra information on baking yeast bread in a bread machine or using the mixer method.

Reheat under the broiler to enjoy crisp focaccia.

Can't decide which topping to make? Make a different topping for each pan.

Substitute any type of bean flour for the pea flour.

Focaccia can be reheated in just a few minutes in a toaster oven set to 375°F (190°C).

Two 9-inch (2.5 L) square baking pans, lightly greased

²/₃ cup	amaranth flour	150 mL
½ cup	pea flour	125 mL
⅓ cup	potato starch	75 mL
¼ cup	tapioca starch	50 mL
1 tsp	granulated sugar	5 mL
2 tsp	xanthan gum	10 mL
1 tbsp	bread machine or instant yeast	15 mL
¾ tsp	salt	4 mL
1½ cups	water	375 mL
1 tbsp	extra-virgin olive oil	15 mL
1 tsp	cider vinegar	5 mL
	Topping mixture (see recipes, pages 81–82)	

Bread Machine Method

1. In a large bowl or plastic bag, combine amaranth flour, pea flour, potato starch, tapioca starch, sugar, xanthan gum, yeast and salt. Mix well and set aside.

2. Pour water, olive oil and vinegar into the bread machine baking pan. Select the **Dough Cycle**. Allow the liquids to mix until combined. As the bread machine is mixing, gradually add the dry ingredients, scraping bottom and sides of pan with a rubber spatula. Try to incorporate all the dry ingredients within 1 to 2 minutes. Stop bread machine as soon as the kneading portion of the cycle is complete. Do not let bread machine finish the cycle.

Mixer Method

1. In a large bowl or plastic bag, combine amaranth flour, pea flour, potato starch, tapioca starch, sugar, xanthan gum, yeast and salt. Mix well and set aside.

2. In a separate bowl, using a heavy-duty electric mixer with paddle attachment, combine water, olive oil and vinegar. With the mixer on its lowest speed, slowly add the dry ingredients until combined. Stop the machine and scrape the bottom and sides of the bowl with a rubber spatula. With the mixer on medium speed, beat for 4 minutes.

For Both Methods

3. Gently transfer the dough to prepared pans, leaving the tops rough and uneven. Do not smooth. Let rise, uncovered, in a warm, draft-free place for 30 minutes. Meanwhile, preheat oven to 400°F (200°C)

4. Bake in preheated oven for 10 minutes, or until bottom is golden.

5. Cover with preferred topping mixture. Bake for another 20 to 25 minutes, or until top is golden. Remove from pans immediately. Serve hot.

Triple-Cheese Focaccia Topping

<table>
<tr><td>2</td><td>cloves garlic, minced</td><td>2</td></tr>
<tr><td>1 tbsp</td><td>extra-virgin olive oil</td><td>15 mL</td></tr>
<tr><td>1 tbsp</td><td>dried basil</td><td>15 mL</td></tr>
<tr><td>1/2 cup</td><td>shredded Asiago cheese</td><td>125 mL</td></tr>
<tr><td>1/2 cup</td><td>shredded mozzarella cheese</td><td>125 mL</td></tr>
<tr><td>1/4 cup</td><td>freshly grated Parmesan cheese</td><td>50 mL</td></tr>
<tr><td>3/4 cup</td><td>GF salsa</td><td>175 mL</td></tr>
</table>

MAKES ENOUGH TOPPING FOR ONE 9-INCH (2.5 L) SQUARE BAKING PAN

A trio of cheeses sprinkled over focaccia dough creates the perfect bread to accompany gazpacho on a hot summer's day.

Tips

Use the amount of cheese stated in the recipe: too much results in a greasy focaccia.

Substitute your favorite lower-fat varieties for the cheeses.

Substitute Black Bean Salsa (see recipe, page 102) for the prepared salsa.

1. In a small bowl, combine garlic, olive oil and basil; let stand while focaccia rises.

2. In another small bowl, combine Asiago, mozzarella and Parmesan. Set aside.

3. Drizzle garlic-oil mixture over the partially cooked focaccia. Top with salsa and cheese mixture.

Mediterranean Focaccia Topping

*Top focaccia with sweet
onions, slowly caramelized
in a very small amount
of olive oil until golden.*

Tip

No need for extra oil: add
1 tbsp (15 mL) white
wine or water to keep
onions from sticking.

1 tbsp	extra-virgin olive oil	15 mL
2 cups	sliced Vidalia or other sweet onions	500 mL
2 tbsp	snipped fresh thyme	25 mL
1 tbsp	balsamic vinegar	15 mL
12	kalamata olives, pitted and sliced	12
1/2 cup	crumbled feta cheese	125 mL

1. In a skillet, heat olive oil over medium-low heat.
   Add onions, stirring frequently, until tender and deep
   golden brown, about 20 minutes. Remove from heat.
   Stir in thyme and vinegar. Cool slightly. Spoon over
   the partially cooked focaccia. Sprinkle with olives
   and feta.

Variation
Add 1/2 cup (125 mL) snipped sun-dried tomatoes.

Parmesan Walnut Focaccia Topping

*Walnuts with freshly
grated Parmesan cheese is
a combination of flavors
sure to please.*

Tips
Store walnuts in the
refrigerator and taste for
freshness before using.

Pine nuts can be
substituted for walnuts
and Romano or Asiago
cheese for the Parmesan.

2	cloves garlic, minced	2
1 to 2 tbsp	extra-virgin olive oil	15 to 25 mL
1/2 cup	finely chopped walnuts	125 mL
3 tbsp	freshly grated Parmesan cheese	45 mL

1. In a small bowl, combine garlic and olive oil; let stand
   while focaccia rises. Drizzle over the partially cooked
   focaccia.
2. Sprinkle with walnuts and Parmesan.

Is Your Diet High in Fiber?

Most GF flours, starches and purchased, prepared products are low in fiber, yet studies have proven fiber's importance and that most of us don't get enough fiber in our diets. Here are some ways to increase fiber while enhancing flavor:

1. Choose flours that are higher in fiber than white rice flour, including amaranth, buckwheat, quinoa, whole bean and chickpea (garbanzo bean).

2. Purchase brown rice in place of white rice and brown rice flour in place of white rice flour.

3. Enjoy high-fiber fruits, including berries, figs, pears and apples. Try Figgy Apple Muffins or Loaf (page 50), Blueberry Almond Dessert (page 160) and Pecan Pear Muffins or Loaf (page 51). When possible, leave the skin on apples, pears, and peaches. Choose raw fruit over juice.

4. Leave the peel on vegetables such as zucchini and cucumber when eating raw or cooked, chopping for a salad or baking in quick breads, muffins or cakes.

5. Add nuts, dried fruit and seeds to salads, breads, cakes and pies. Try Carrot Apple Energy Bars (page 43) and Henk's Flax Bread (pages 78–79). Remember to crack or grind flaxseed to enable the body to absorb the nutrients.

6. Purchase high-fiber GF cereals for breakfast, crumb crusts and toppings.

7. Plan to use peas, beans, quinoa and lentils for dips, salads and pilafs. Serve Halibut Steaks with Black Bean Salsa (page 102) with a generous serving of Savory Vegetarian Quinoa Pilaf (page 103).

8. Snack on roasted pumpkin seeds, sunflower seeds and toasted almonds. Make your own granola (Linda's Granola, page 44).

Sun-dried Tomato Ciabatta

A traditional ciabatta with a modern twist. Sun-dried tomatoes, Parmesan cheese and fresh rosemary take this Italian flatbread a step above the ordinary.

Tips

To ensure success, see page 67 for extra information on baking yeast bread in a bread machine or using the mixer method.

We like this ciabatta best served hot out of the oven.

Break this bread into pieces to serve with soups or salads.

9-inch (23 cm) round baking pan, lightly floured with sweet rice flour

1/2 cup	brown rice flour	125 mL
1/2 cup	whole bean flour	125 mL
1/3 cup	tapioca starch	75 mL
2 tbsp	granulated sugar	25 mL
2 tsp	xanthan gum	10 mL
2 tbsp	bread machine or instant yeast	25 mL
1/4 tsp	salt	1 mL
1 cup	freshly grated Parmesan cheese	250 mL
1/4 cup	chopped fresh rosemary	50 mL
3/4 cup	water	175 mL
1/4 cup	extra-virgin olive oil	50 mL
1 tsp	cider vinegar	5 mL
2	eggs	2
2	cloves garlic, minced	2
2/3 cup	snipped sun-dried tomatoes	150 mL
	Sweet rice flour	

Bread Machine Method

1. In a large bowl or plastic bag, combine brown rice flour, whole bean flour, tapioca starch, sugar, xanthan gum, yeast, salt, Parmesan cheese and rosemary. Mix well and set aside.

2. Pour water, olive oil and vinegar into the bread machine baking pan. Add eggs, garlic and sun-dried tomatoes. Select the **Dough Cycle**. Allow the liquids to mix until combined. As the bread machine is mixing, gradually add the dry ingredients, scraping bottom and sides of pan with a rubber spatula. Try to incorporate all the dry ingredients within 1 to 2 minutes. Allow the bread machine to complete the cycle.

Mixer Method

1. In a large bowl or plastic bag, combine brown rice flour, whole bean flour, tapioca starch, sugar, xanthan gum, yeast, salt, Parmesan cheese and rosemary. Mix well and set aside.

2. In a separate bowl, using a heavy-duty electric mixer with paddle attachment, combine water, olive oil, vinegar, eggs, garlic and sun-dried tomatoes until well blended. With the mixer on its lowest speed, slowly add the dry ingredients until combined. Stop the machine and scrape the bottom and sides of the bowl with a rubber spatula. With the mixer on medium speed, beat for 4 minutes.

For Both Methods

3. Immediately transfer dough to prepared pan and spread evenly. Generously dust top with sweet rice flour. With well-floured fingers, make deep indents all over the dough, making sure to press all the way down to the pan. Let rise, uncovered, in a warm, draft-free place for 60 minutes, or until almost double in volume. Meanwhile, preheat oven to 425°F (220°C).

4. Bake in preheated oven for 20 to 25 minutes, or until bread is golden and sounds hollow when top is tapped. Remove from pan immediately and serve.

Variation

Substitute 2 to 3 tbsp (25 to 45 mL) dried basil or oregano for the fresh rosemary and sprinkle the risen dough with 2 tbsp (25 mL) freshly grated Parmesan cheese.

Egg-Free, Corn-Free, Lactose-Free Brown Bread

The perfect sandwich bread! Just add shaved roast beef, a leaf of romaine and a hint of mustard. It carries well for a tasty lunch.

Tips

Slice this or any bread with an electric knife for thin, even sandwich slices.

For information about egg replacer, see Ingredient Glossary, page 175.

For a milder-flavored bread, substitute 2 tbsp (25 mL) packed brown sugar for the molasses.

The rice bran can be replaced by an equal amount of brown or white rice flour.

9- by 5-inch (2 L) loaf pan, lightly greased

1¼ cups	brown rice flour	300 mL
½ cup	sorghum flour	125 mL
½ cup	rice bran	125 mL
¼ cup	tapioca starch	50 mL
1 tbsp	powdered egg replacer	15 mL
1 tbsp	xanthan gum	15 mL
1 tbsp	bread machine or instant yeast	15 mL
1¼ tsp	salt	6 mL
1⅓ cups	water	325 mL
2 tbsp	vegetable oil	25 mL
2 tbsp	liquid honey	25 mL
1 tbsp	fancy molasses	15 mL
1 tsp	cider vinegar	5 mL

1. In a large bowl or plastic bag, combine brown rice flour, sorghum flour, rice bran, tapioca starch, egg replacer, xanthan gum, yeast and salt. Mix well and set aside.

2. In a separate bowl, using a heavy-duty electric mixer with paddle attachment, combine water, oil, honey, molasses and vinegar until well blended. With the mixer on its lowest speed, slowly add the dry ingredients until combined. Stop the machine and scrape the bottom and sides of the bowl with a rubber spatula. With the mixer on medium speed, beat for 4 minutes.

3. Spoon into prepared pan. Let rise, uncovered, in a warm, draft-free place for 60 to 75 minutes, or until dough has risen to the top of the pan. Meanwhile, preheat oven to 350°F (180°C).

4. Bake for 35 to 45 minutes, or until loaf sounds hollow when tapped on the bottom. Remove from the pan immediately and let cool completely on a rack.

Egg-Free, Corn-Free, Lactose-Free White Bread

MAKES 1 LOAF

We know you'll enjoy this moist, all-purpose yeast bread, whether for sandwiches or to accompany your favorite salad.

Tips

Thoroughly mix the dry ingredients before adding them to the liquids — they are powder-fine and can clump together.

Use any leftovers to make bread crumbs (see Techniques Glossary, page 179).

To make your own almond flour, see Techniques Glossary, page 181, under Nut flour.

For information about egg replacer, see Ingredient Glossary, page 175.

9- by 5-inch (2 L) loaf pan, lightly greased

1¾ cups	brown rice flour	425 mL
¼ cup	almond flour	50 mL
½ cup	potato starch	125 mL
¼ cup	tapioca starch	50 mL
1 tbsp	powdered egg replacer	15 mL
2 tbsp	granulated sugar	25 mL
2½ tsp	xanthan gum	12 mL
2 tsp	bread machine or instant yeast	10 mL
1¼ tsp	salt	6 mL
1⅓ cups	water	325 mL
2 tbsp	vegetable oil	25 mL
2 tsp	cider vinegar	10 mL

1. In a large bowl or plastic bag, combine rice flour, almond flour, potato starch, tapioca starch, egg replacer, sugar, xanthan gum, yeast and salt. Mix well and set aside.

2. In a separate bowl, using a heavy-duty electric mixer with paddle attachment, combine water, oil and vinegar until well blended. With the mixer on its lowest speed, slowly add the dry ingredients until combined. Stop the machine and scrape the bottom and sides of the bowl with a rubber spatula. With the mixer on medium speed, beat for 4 minutes.

3. Spoon into prepared pan. Let rise, uncovered, in a warm, draft-free place for 60 to 75 minutes, or until dough has risen to the top of the pan. Meanwhile, preheat oven to 350°F (180°C).

4. Bake for 35 to 45 minutes, or until loaf sounds hollow when tapped on the bottom. Remove from the pan immediately and let cool completely on a rack.

Chocolate Fig Panettone

More like chocolate cake than bread, these mini-loaves are rich, sweet and brimming with fruit! Panettone originated in Milan, Italy, where it is served at Christmas and Easter, and for weddings and christenings. Break with tradition and try our modern flavor combination.

Tips

Thoroughly mix the dry ingredients before adding them to the liquids — they are powder-fine and can clump together.

Purchase 4 to 5 medium-sized figs for the ¹/₂ cup (125 mL) chopped figs.

Use a coffee grinder (reserved for spices) to crush the anise seed.

Three 5¹/₂- by 3-inch (500 mL) mini-loaf pans, lightly greased

³/₄ cup	amaranth flour	175 mL
¹/₂ cup	brown rice flour	125 mL
¹/₂ cup	potato starch	125 mL
¹/₄ cup	tapioca starch	50 mL
¹/₂ cup	granulated sugar	125 mL
¹/₄ cup	nonfat (skim) milk powder	50 mL
¹/₄ cup	unsweetened cocoa powder, sifted	50 mL
1 tbsp	xanthan gum	15 mL
1 tbsp	bread machine or instant yeast	15 mL
1¹/₄ tsp	salt	6 mL
1 tsp	crushed anise seed	5 mL
2	eggs	2
2	egg whites	2
1 cup	water	250 mL
¹/₄ cup	vegetable oil	50 mL
2 tsp	cider vinegar	10 mL
¹/₂ cup	chopped dried figs	125 mL
¹/₂ cup	chocolate chips	125 mL
¹/₂ cup	raisins	125 mL

1. In a large bowl or plastic bag, combine amaranth flour, brown rice flour, potato starch, tapioca starch, sugar, milk powder, cocoa powder, xanthan gum, yeast, salt and anise seed. Mix well and set aside.

Bake in single-use mini-pans, wrap in festive cellophane and tie with a bow to give as gifts.

For a lactose-free loaf, omit the milk powder.

2. In a separate bowl, using a heavy-duty electric mixer with paddle attachment, combine eggs, egg whites, water, oil and vinegar until well blended. With the mixer on its lowest speed, slowly add the dry ingredients until combined. Stop the machine and scrape the bottom and sides of the bowl with a rubber spatula. With the mixer on medium speed, beat for 4 minutes. Stir in figs, chocolate chips and raisins.

3. Spoon into prepared pans. Let rise, uncovered, in a warm, draft-free place for 60 to 75 minutes, or until dough has risen to the top of the pans. Meanwhile, preheat oven to 350°F (180°C).

4. Bake for 30 to 35 minutes, or until loaves sound hollow when tapped on the bottom. Remove from the pans immediately and let cool completely on a rack.

Variation
Substitute an equal amount of candied mixed peel and candied citron for the figs and chocolate chips.

Orange Marmalade

MAKES 4 CUPS (1 L)

Looking for a change of spreads for your morning toast? You'll want to make extra so you can take a jar of this delicious marmalade with you the next time you visit friends.

Tips

Handle the marmalade carefully — it is still extremely hot after cooling for 30 minutes in the bread machine.

2 to 3 medium carrots yield $1^1/_2$ cups (375 mL) grated.

If you don't have a **Jam Cycle** on your bread machine, try mixing ingredients for 5 to 6 minutes on the **Basic Cycle**. Turn off the bread machine, then restart it and select the **Bake Cycle**.

You can use Valencia oranges, but for a stronger flavor wait for the Seville orange harvest.

2	oranges	2
1	lemon	1
$^1/_2$ cup	water	125 mL
$2^1/_2$ cups	granulated sugar	625 mL
$1^1/_2$ cups	grated carrots	375 mL

1. Wash and scrub the peels of oranges and lemon. Cut each into eight pieces and remove tough center membranes and seeds.
2. In a food processor fitted with a metal blade, pulse oranges and lemon until coarsely chopped.
3. Pour water into bread machine baking pan; add sugar, carrots, oranges and lemon. Insert pan into oven chamber and select the **Jam Cycle**.
4. At the end of the cycle, carefully open the lid of the bread machine and let baking pan remain in the machine for 30 minutes.
5. Remove baking pan carefully and ladle marmalade into sterilized jars, leaving $^1/_4$-inch (0.5 cm) headspace. Store in the refrigerator for up to 4 weeks, freeze for up to 4 months or process in a water bath (see Techniques Glossary, page 181) for 5 minutes to preserve jam so it is shelf stable.

Variation

For thicker marmalade, add 2 to 3 tsp (10 to 15 mL) "light" pectin crystals with the fruit.

What's for Dinner?

Here are some suggestions to solve the age-old question "What's for dinner?"

Chicken Vegetable Bundles with Mushroom Sauce

This dish is tasty enough to serve to company, but simple enough to make for your family any weeknight.

Tips

If you don't have a deep skillet, use an electric frying pan, a Dutch oven or a large covered saucepan.

Using evaporated milk instead of regular milk doubles the calcium.

See Techniques Glossary, page 179, for information on testing doneness with a digital instant-read thermometer.

For a richer flavor, use a variety of mushrooms. You can include shiitake, cremini (firmer and with a stronger flavor than a regular white button), portobellini or portobello (mature cremini with a strong, concentrated flavor). There are two portobello mushroom caps in 8 oz (250 g).

9- to 10-inch (23 to 25 cm) skillet, 2 inches (5 cm) deep

4	skinless boneless chicken breasts	4
16	snow peas	16
1	small zucchini, cut into 1/2-inch (1 cm) strips	1
1	small sweet potato, cut into 1/2-inch (1 cm) strips	1
1 tbsp	vegetable oil	15 mL
2	cloves garlic, finely chopped	2
1	medium onion, halved lengthwise and thickly sliced	1
8 oz	mushrooms, sliced	250 g
1 tsp	dried sage	5 mL
1/4 tsp	salt	1 mL
	Freshly ground white pepper	
1	can (14 oz/385 mL) 2% evaporated milk	1
3 tbsp	cornstarch	45 mL
2 tbsp	water	25 mL
1 tsp	freshly squeezed lemon juice	5 mL
	Cooked rice noodles, GF pasta or rice	

1. With a sharp knife, cut chicken breasts lengthwise almost in half, being careful not to cut all the way through. Open and flatten. Place one quarter of the snow peas, zucchini strips and sweet potato strips on half of each chicken breast. Fold the remaining half of the chicken breast over the vegetables.

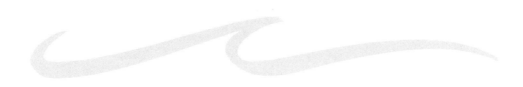

Mushrooms can be stored in the refrigerator in a paper bag for up to 3 to 4 days.

Substitute fresh asparagus, green beans, red pepper, winter squash or turnip for any of the vegetables.

2. In a large nonstick skillet, heat oil over medium-low heat. Cook garlic, onion, mushrooms, sage, salt and pepper to taste until vegetables are tender; stirring occasionally. Whisk in evaporated milk.

3. Add chicken, seam side down, and bring to a boil. Cover, reduce heat and simmer gently for approximately 25 to 30 minutes, or until digital instant-read thermometer registers 170°F (78°C) and chicken is no longer pink inside. Remove chicken to a serving platter and keep warm.

4. In a small bowl, combine cornstarch and water; add to skillet and cook, stirring, for 2 to 3 minutes, or until thickened. Stir in lemon juice.

5. Serve the chicken and mushroom sauce over hot rice noodles, gluten-free pasta or rice.

Ten-Minute Pasta Dinner

In a hurry again? Want to make dinner without stopping at a grocery store on the way home from work? Chances are you have every ingredient you need to make this in the cupboard and freezer.

Tips

Shrimp become rubbery when overcooked. They are cooked when they curl, turn pink and are firm to the touch.

Select from the many varieties of mixed frozen vegetables on the market today — Japanese Mix, California Combo, Asian or Thai Stir-Fry, Mexican- or Spanish-style or an Orleans mix.

For a richer, thicker sauce, substitute a 23-oz (680 mL) can of GF Roasted Garlic and Herb Pasta Sauce for the tomatoes.

1½ cups	GF pasta	375 mL
4 cups	mixed frozen vegetables	1 L
12 oz	frozen raw extra-large or jumbo shrimp, thawed	340 g
1	can (28 oz/796 mL) GF diced tomatoes with herbs and spices	1
2 tsp	dried basil	10 mL
	Freshly grated Parmesan cheese	

1. In a large saucepan of boiling water, cook pasta according to package directions, or until just tender. Drain well and rinse in cold water. Set aside.
2. In a separate saucepan, cook frozen vegetables according to package directions. Add shrimp for the last 2 minutes, until shrimp turn pink.
3. Meanwhile, add tomatoes and basil to empty pasta saucepan and heat over medium-high heat until bubbling. Add cooked pasta and vegetable mixture and heat just until steaming.
4. Ladle into a serving bowl and sprinkle with Parmesan cheese.

Variations

Substitute 2 cups (500 mL) cooked chicken or ham, cut into cubes or strips, for the shrimp. Add during the last 2 minutes.

Substitute mussels for shrimp and steam until they open, about 5 to 8 minutes. Discard any mussels that do not open.

Fresh Tomato-Leek Sauce with Sea Scallops

Succulent tender sea scallops, nestled in a bed of gluten-free pasta and accented with a colorful Fresh Tomato-Leek Sauce.

Tips

1 cup (250 mL) snow peas or tender pea pods weighs about 4 oz (125 g).

See Techniques Glossary, page 180, for information about cleaning leeks.

There are approximately 12 sea scallops in 8 oz (250 g).

Vary the herb according to your preference. Try basil or dill.

Substitute GF chicken stock for the white wine.

1 cup	snow peas	250 mL
2 tbsp	extra-virgin olive oil	25 mL
2	leeks, white and light green parts only, cut into 1-inch (2.5 cm) slices	2
2	cloves garlic, minced	2
2	tomatoes, seeded and chopped	2
8 oz	scallops	250 g
1/4 cup	snipped fresh cilantro	50 mL
1/4 cup	dry white wine	50 mL
	Salt and freshly ground black pepper	
	Cooked rice or GF pasta	

1. Trim tops and remove strings from snow peas. Set aside.
2. In a large saucepan, heat olive oil over medium heat. Add snow peas, leeks and garlic and cook, stirring, for 5 minutes, or until tender-crisp. Add tomatoes, scallops, cilantro and wine. Reduce heat to medium-low and simmer for 3 to 5 minutes, or until scallops are opaque. Season with salt and pepper to taste.
3. Serve over hot rice or gluten-free pasta.

Variation

Shrimp, monkfish, clams or mussels, or a combination, can be substituted for the scallops.

Broccoli Cilantro Pesto with Pasta

Make good use of homegrown produce when it's at its best. Turn it into a meal by serving it with Italian Sausage Patties (see recipe, page 97) and fresh grape tomatoes.

Tips

4 cups (1 L) of broccoli florets weigh 1 pound (500 g).

Add more GF chicken stock if the pesto seems too thick.

Make lots of pesto during the summer, when herbs are plentiful, and freeze in small quantities.

Vary the herbs and the amounts used.

4 cups	broccoli florets	1 L
1	clove garlic, minced	1
½ cup	snipped fresh cilantro	125 mL
¼ cup	snipped fresh basil	50 mL
¼ cup	freshly grated Parmesan cheese	50 mL
¼ cup	extra-virgin olive oil	50 mL
¼ cup	GF chicken stock	50 mL
¼ tsp	salt	1 mL
	Cooked GF pasta	

1. In a glass bowl, microwave broccoli florets, covered, on High (100%) for 3 to 5 minutes, or until tender-crisp, or steam in a vegetable steamer until tender-crisp.
2. In a food processor fitted with a metal blade, combine broccoli, garlic, cilantro, basil, Parmesan, olive oil, stock and salt. Process until coarsely chopped.
3. Toss pesto with hot cooked GF pasta.

Italian Sausage Patties

Serve these spicy meat patties over pasta, in a pesto sauce or with a mild tomato sauce. Make ahead and freeze for up to 3 months for a last-minute supper or snack.

Tips

If you use an indoor contact grill, there is no need to turn the patties. Cooking time will be much shorter; check the manufacturer's instructions.

See Equipment Glossary, page 172, for more information on meat thermometers.

For a stronger flavor, substitute caraway or anise seed for the fennel.

Barbecue, grill or broiler, preheated

1 lb	lean ground beef	500 g
3	cloves garlic, minced	3
2 tsp	fennel seeds	10 mL
1 tsp	hot pepper flakes	5 mL
¾ tsp	salt	4 mL
½ tsp	freshly ground black pepper	2 mL
¼ tsp	cayenne pepper (optional)	1 mL

1. In a medium bowl, using a fork, gently combine beef, garlic, fennel seeds, hot pepper flakes, salt, pepper and cayenne pepper, if using. Form into 12 patties, 2 inches (5 cm) in diameter.

2. On preheated barbecue, grill patties for 2 to 3 minutes, turning only once, until meat thermometer registers 160°F (70°C) and patties are no longer pink inside.

Variations

Substitute ground veal, pork, chicken or turkey for the ground beef.

Make into meatballs. Bake on a baking sheet at 400°F (200°C) for 15 to 20 minutes, or until no longer pink in the center.

Sesame Thai Beef

We first tasted this dish in a restaurant in Toronto. Joyce Parslow of the Canadian Beef Information Centre was kind enough to provide us with a recipe, which we have adapted for you. This is the perfect dish for a dinner party at which everyone contributes to the preparation of the meal.

Tips

You can use either a mandoline with the julienne $^1/_{16}$- to $^1/_4$-inch (2 to 5 mm) blade or a sharp knife to cut vegetables into matchstick-size pieces. This means sliced paper-thin, as the only cooking is from the hot stock in individual bowls.

To make slicing easier, place the beef steak in the freezer until it's almost firm. For thin slices, be sure knife is sharp and slice across the grain.

Always discard leftover mixtures used for marinating raw meats, fish and poultry.

SESAME MARINADE

$^1/_4$ cup	minced green onions	50 mL
$^1/_4$ cup	vegetable oil	50 mL
$^1/_4$ cup	dry sherry	50 mL
2 tbsp	toasted sesame seeds	25 mL
2 tbsp	sesame oil	25 mL
1 tbsp	minced gingerroot	15 mL
1 tbsp	GF soy sauce	15 mL
1 tbsp	minced garlic	15 mL
$1^1/_2$ tsp	sambal oelek	7 mL
1 lb	boneless beef strip loin (top loin) grilling steak, sliced into $^1/_8$-inch (3 mm) strips	500 g

NOODLE BOWL

5 cups	water	1.25 L
$^1/_2$ cup	sliced onions	125 mL
2 tbsp	GF chicken or vegetable stock powder	25 mL
2 tbsp	reserved sesame marinade	25 mL
$1^1/_2$ tsp	thinly sliced gingerroot	7 mL
$1^1/_2$ tsp	thinly sliced garlic	7 mL
7 oz	GF rice vermicelli or rice sticks, cooked	200 g
2 cups	shredded bok choy	500 mL
$1^1/_2$ cups	julienned red bell peppers	375 mL
1 cup	julienned carrots	250 mL
$^3/_4$ cup	julienned green onions	175 mL
2 tbsp	snipped fresh cilantro	25 mL

1. *Prepare the sesame marinade:* In a resealable plastic freezer bag set in a bowl, combine green onions, vegetable oil, sherry, sesame seeds, sesame oil, gingerroot, soy sauce, garlic and sambal oelek. Set aside 2 tbsp (25 mL) of the marinade for the noodle bowl.

To learn more about sambal oelek, see Ingredient Glossary, page 177. It can be found in the Asian section of large chain grocery stores or at Asian grocers and Dutch delicatessens.

Use an equal amount of hot pepper flakes if sambal oelek is not available.

Try a flank steak instead of the strip loin steak.

Substitute unsweetened apple juice or water for the sherry.

Substitute 5 cups (1.25 L) homemade or commercial GF chicken or vegetable stock for the stock powder and water.

2. Add beef strips to remaining marinade, seal bag and refrigerate for at least 6 hours or overnight.

3. *Prepare the noodle bowl:* In a large saucepan, over high heat, combine water, onions, stock powder, reserved marinade, gingerroot and garlic and bring to a boil. Reduce heat and simmer for 5 minutes. Add noodles and boil for 1 minute, until hot. Drain, reserving stock mixture. Return stock to a boil and continue to gently simmer. Set noodles in a strainer over simmering stock to keep warm.

4. Heat a large nonstick skillet or wok over high heat until very hot. Drain beef strips from marinade, discarding marinade, and add to skillet. Cook, in batches, as necessary, for 1 minute on each side.

5. *To serve:* Divide bok choy, red peppers, carrots, green onions, noodles and beef among 4 large soup or pasta bowls. Pour 1 cup (250 mL) reserved boiling stock mixture over each. Garnish with cilantro.

Grilled Salmon and Roasted Peppers with Fusilli

What an delicious way to increase your omega-3 fatty acids.

Tips

Roast peppers on the barbecue the next time you have it fired up. To heighten the flavor of the roasted peppers, be sure to cook them long enough for the skins to appear burnt and begin to flake off.

In the fall, when peppers are plentiful, roast extra and freeze them, so you'll have them available all winter long.

Salmon can be grilled directly from the freezer. Increase the cooking time to 20 minutes per inch (2.5 cm) of thickness. Turn only once.

If you use an indoor contact grill, there's no need to turn the fish, as both sides cook at once. Cooking time for both peppers and fish may be shorter; check the manufacturer's instructions.

Barbeque, grill or broiler, preheated

2	large red bell peppers	2
1	large orange bell pepper	1
1	large yellow bell pepper	1
4	salmon fillets, with skin, 1 inch (2.5 cm) thick (each 6 oz/175 g)	4
2 tsp	extra-virgin olive oil	10 mL
3	cloves garlic, thickly sliced	3
6 oz	GF fusilli noodles	175 g
1/4 cup	toasted pine nuts	50 mL
	Lemon wedges	

SAUCE

1	can (14 oz/385 mL) 2% evaporated milk	1
1/3 cup	freshly grated Parmesan cheese	75 mL
2 tbsp	cornstarch	25 mL
5 oz	baby spinach	150 g
1/2 tsp	salt	2 mL
1/4 tsp	freshly ground black pepper	1 mL
1/2 tsp	freshly squeezed lemon juice	2 mL

1. Cut peppers in half and remove the stems, seeds and white membrane. Place peppers on preheated barbecue or on a baking sheet under broiler, cut side down, and grill or broil for 15 to 20 minutes, or until skin blisters, becomes scorched and blackens. Place peppers in a small glass bowl, cover tightly with plastic wrap and let stand for 15 minutes. When peppers have cooled slightly, peel off blackened skin. Cut each half into six strips.

2. Brush both sides of each salmon fillet with olive oil. Grill or broil on a broiler pan, turning once, for about 10 minutes per inch (2.5 cm) of thickness, or until fish is opaque and flakes easily when tested with a fork.

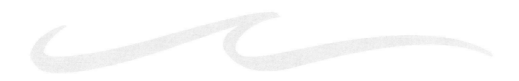

See Techniques Glossary, page 181, under Nuts, for tips on toasting pine nuts.

Substitute any firm fish fillet for the salmon.

Substitute an equal quantity of soy nuts for the pine nuts.

We used wild rice fusilli, but you can use GF pasta of any shape or flavor in this recipe.

3. Meanwhile, in a large saucepan of gently boiling water, cook garlic and fusilli according to pasta package directions. Drain; discard garlic.

4. *Prepare the sauce:* In a large saucepan, over medium heat, whisk together evaporated milk, Parmesan and cornstarch. Bring to a simmer; add spinach, salt and pepper. Simmer until spinach is wilted, about 3 minutes. Stir in pepper strips, cooked pasta and lemon juice. Heat thoroughly.

5. Spoon onto a large serving platter and top with salmon and toasted pine nuts. Garnish with wedges of lemon.

Lemon Dill Sauce

This creamy sauce is delicious served with grilled salmon, steamed asparagus or roasted baby carrots.

Tips
Use any type of milk: skim (nonfat), 1%, 2%, or homogenized (whole) milk.

Substitute whole bean flour for the amaranth flour.

2 tbsp	butter	25 mL
3 tbsp	amaranth flour	45 mL
1 cup	milk	250 mL
1 tbsp	freshly squeezed lemon juice	15 mL
¹⁄₂ tsp	dried dillweed	2 mL
	Salt and freshly ground white pepper	

1. In a saucepan, melt butter over medium heat. Stir in amaranth flour and mix just until blended. Gradually add milk, stirring constantly. Bring to a boil and cook, stirring constantly, for 5 to 7 minutes, or until thickened. Stir in lemon juice and dillweed and season to taste with salt and pepper.

Variation

For a brown sauce, brown the amaranth flour and butter mixture for 3 to 5 minutes and substitute GF beef stock for the milk. Omit the lemon and dillweed.

Halibut Steaks with Black Bean Salsa

Looking for a quick, nutritious supper for a busy weeknight? Nothing cooks faster than fish.

Tip

Grill halibut directly from the freezer. Increase cooking time to 20 minutes per inch (2.5 cm) of thickness. Turn only once.

Barbecue, grill or broiler, preheated

2 tbsp	freshly squeezed lemon juice	25 mL
1 tbsp	extra-virgin olive oil	15 mL
4	halibut steaks (each 6 oz/175 g)	4
	Black Bean Salsa (see recipe, below)	

1. In a shallow glass dish, whisk together lemon juice and olive oil. Add fish and turn to coat.
2. Place fish on preheated barbecue, close lid and grill (or broil on a broiler pan) for about 10 minutes per inch (2.5 cm) of thickness, turning once, until fish is opaque and flakes easily when tested with a fork.
3. Spoon Black Bean Salsa over the halibut and serve.

Black Bean Salsa

MAKES 3 CUPS (750 mL)

Tips

If canned black beans are not available, cook 1 cup (250 mL) dried black beans. For instructions, see Techniques Glossary, page 179.

Substitute a canned bean salad mix for the black beans.

Add 1 cup (250 mL) well-drained whole corn kernels, either canned or frozen.

1	can (19 oz/540 mL) black beans, rinsed and drained	1
2	green onions, thinly sliced	2
1	large red bell pepper, finely chopped	1
1	large tomato, seeded and finely chopped	1
¼ cup	snipped fresh cilantro	50 mL
2 tbsp	extra-virgin olive oil	25 mL
2 tbsp	red wine vinegar	25 mL
1 tbsp	chili powder	15 mL
	Salt and freshly ground black pepper	

1. In a large bowl, combine black beans, green onions, bell pepper, tomato, cilantro, olive oil, vinegar and chili powder. Season to taste with salt and pepper.
2. Cover and refrigerate for a minimum of 6 hours or overnight to allow flavors to develop and blend. Refrigerate for up to 2 weeks.

Savory Vegetarian Quinoa Pilaf

This delicious vegetarian dish is dotted with multicolored chunks of nutritious vegetables.

Tips

Quinoa is cooked when grains turn from white to transparent and the tiny spiral-like germ is separated.

For a richer, robust pilaf, substitute GF beef or GF chicken stock for the vegetable stock.

2 tsp	extra-virgin olive oil	10 mL
1	stalk celery, diced	1
1	medium carrot, coarsely chopped	1
1/2	small onion, coarsely chopped	1/2
1 1/2 cups	GF vegetable stock	375 mL
1/2 cup	quinoa	125 mL
1 tsp	dried basil	5 mL
	Salt and freshly ground black pepper	
1	red bell pepper, cut into 1/2-inch (1 cm) cubes	1
1	orange bell pepper, cut into 1/2-inch (1 cm) cubes	1
2	green onions, green tops only, chopped	2

1. In a large saucepan, heat olive oil over medium-low heat. Add celery, carrot and onion and cook, stirring frequently, for about 8 to 10 minutes, or until tender. Add stock, quinoa and basil and bring to a boil.

2. Reduce heat to low; cover and simmer for 18 to 20 minutes, or until water is absorbed and quinoa is tender. Season to taste with salt and pepper. Stir in red and orange peppers and green onion; let stand, covered, for 2 to 3 minutes.

Variation

Add small broccoli florets with the bell peppers. They add a tender-crisp texture.

Quinoa-Stuffed Peppers

This entrée comes to mind in the late summer, when the vegetables are ripe in the garden. We often forget to make it in the winter.

Tips

Assemble early in the day, then refrigerate, covered, to serve for dinner. Allow double the cooking time if cold from the refrigerator.

Sprinkle any remaining stuffing in the bottom of the casserole.

See Techniques Glossary, page 181, for instructions on cooking quinoa.

Substitute brown or wild rice for all or part of the quinoa.

Preheat oven to 400°F (200°C)
10-cup (2.5 L) covered casserole dish

1	large orange bell pepper	1
1	large yellow bell pepper	1
1	tomato, sliced into four thick slices	1
¼ cup	dry white wine	50 mL
1 cup	shredded Swiss cheese	250 mL

STUFFING

8 oz	extra-lean ground beef, turkey or chicken	250 g
½	small onion, chopped	½
½	red bell pepper, chopped	½
1 cup	sliced mushrooms	250 mL
1 tbsp	chopped fresh rosemary	15 mL
1 tbsp	chopped fresh thyme	15 mL
1	tomato, chopped	1
1	small zucchini, chopped	1
1 cup	cooked quinoa	250 mL
¼ tsp	salt	1 mL
¼ tsp	freshly ground black pepper	1 mL

1. Cut orange and yellow peppers in half lengthwise and remove core and seeds. Trim a thin slice off the bottom of each to allow them to lie flat. In the casserole dish, microwave peppers, covered, on High for 3 minutes, or until tender-crisp Let cool to room temperature, covered. Drain and pat dry.

Vary the type of mushrooms — try portobello, cremini, oyster or shiitake.

Substitute 1 cup (250 mL) undrained chopped canned tomatoes for the fresh tomato slices and white wine.

2. *Prepare the stuffing:* Meanwhile, in a large skillet, over medium heat, brown ground beef until no pink remains. Add onion, red pepper, mushrooms, rosemary and thyme; cook, stirring, until onions are translucent, about 3 minutes. Drain off any fat. Add chopped tomato and zucchini and cook, stirring, for 5 minutes. Stir in quinoa, salt and pepper.

3. In the casserole dish, arrange tomato slices and add wine. Set each pepper half, cut side up, on a tomato slice. Fill each pepper half with the beef mixture, mounding the stuffing.

4. Cover and bake in preheated oven for 15 minutes, or until bell peppers are fork-tender. Uncover, top with Swiss cheese and bake, uncovered, for 5 minutes more, or until cheese is melted.

Variation

Stuff zucchini in place of the bell peppers. Acorn squash or mini pumpkins can also be stuffed, but must be fully cooked first.

Savory Stilton Cheesecake

SERVES 8

Serve this make-ahead main dish and enjoy the delightful bursts of flavor — just imagine nippy Stilton combined with fresh herbs from your garden.

Tips

Cheesecake keeps for up to 2 days in the refrigerator. It can also be frozen in an airtight container for up to 2 weeks. We froze wedges individually for a quick dinner for two. Bring to room temperature before serving.

8 oz (250 g) of Stilton cheese yield 1$\frac{1}{2}$ cups (375 mL).

Use the hottest tap water available to fill the roasting pan in the oven to a depth of 1 inch (2.5 cm).

Leaving the cheesecake in the oven after turning it off helps prevent large cracks. Be sure to set a timer, as it is easy to forget.

Preheat oven to 325°F (160°C)
9-inch (23 cm) springform pan, lightly greased

BASE

1$\frac{1}{2}$ cups	fresh GF bread crumbs	375 mL
$\frac{2}{3}$ cup	chopped walnuts	150 mL
2 tbsp	melted butter	25 mL

CHEESECAKE

2	packages (each 8 oz/250 g) cream cheese, softened	2
1 tbsp	Dijon mustard	15 mL
3	eggs	3
1	clove garlic, minced	1
1 cup	plain yogurt	250 mL
$\frac{1}{4}$ cup	freshly grated Parmesan cheese	50 mL
2 tbsp	snipped fresh basil	25 mL
2 tbsp	snipped fresh sage	25 mL
1 tbsp	snipped fresh thyme	15 mL
$\frac{1}{4}$ tsp	freshly ground black pepper	1 mL
1$\frac{1}{2}$ cups	cubed Stilton cheese, ($\frac{1}{4}$-inch/0.5 cm cubes)	375 mL

1. *Prepare the base:* In a large bowl, combine bread crumbs, walnuts and butter. Mix well. Press into prepared pan and bake in preheated oven for 20 minutes to partially cook. Let cool to room temperature. Center springform pan on a large square of foil; press foil up sides of pan.

2. *Prepare the cheesecake:* In a large bowl, using an electric mixer, beat the cream cheese and Dijon mustard until smooth. Add eggs one at a time, beating well after each. Stir in garlic, yogurt, Parmesan, basil, sage, thyme and pepper until combined. Fold in Stilton cheese. Pour over base.

After removing the baked cheesecake from the water bath, set the springform pan in an empty sink to carefully remove the foil. The water may leak out.

See Techniques Glossary, page 179, for information on making GF bread crumbs.

Substitute a lower-fat (but not whipped or spreadable) cream cheese.

Substitute GF Danish blue cheese for the Stilton.

3. Place the foil-wrapped springform pan in a larger roasting pan, and set on oven rack placed in the center of the preheated oven. Pour in enough hot water to fill the larger pan to a depth of 1 inch (2.5 cm). Bake for 70 to 80 minutes, or until center is just set and the blade of a knife comes out clean. Turn oven off and let cheesecake cool in oven for 1 hour (see tip, at left). Carefully remove springform pan from pan of water and remove the foil. Let cool in springform pan on a rack for 30 minutes. Refrigerate until chilled, about 3 hours. Bring to room temperature before serving.

Variation

For a stronger walnut flavor, toast the walnuts before chopping (see Techniques Glossary, page 181, under Nuts) and substitute walnut oil for the melted butter.

Spinach Risotto

Packed with fresh vegetables, our variation of risotto — a northern Italian rice dish — is creamy, yet a light and easy-to-prepare side dish.

Tips

The large quantity of spinach might look like too much, but it wilts down to the correct amount for this recipe.

Serve immediately to keep the creamy texture.

For a creamier, more traditional risotto, increase the amount of liquid and add more as it becomes absorbed. Stir constantly while rice is cooking.

Substitute milk for the GF chicken stock or for both the GF chicken stock and wine.

Substitute a carnaroli or any short-grain rice for the Arborio rice.

2 tsp	extra-virgin olive oil	10 mL
2	cloves garlic, minced	2
2	celery stalks, chopped	2
1	medium onion, chopped	1
1	carrot, diced	1
1 cup	Arborio rice	250 mL
1 1/2 cups	GF chicken stock	375 mL
1/2 cup	dry white wine	125 mL
10 oz	baby spinach	300 g
1	small zucchini, chopped	1
1/4 cup	freshly grated Parmesan cheese	50 mL
	Salt, pepper and dried dillweed or grated nutmeg	

1. In a large saucepan, heat olive oil over medium heat. Add garlic, celery, onion, carrot and rice. Cook, stirring, for 5 to 7 minutes, or until vegetables are softened. Stir in stock and wine and bring to a boil over high heat.

2. Reduce heat to medium-low and simmer, covered, for 20 minutes, or until all liquid is absorbed. Stir in spinach, zucchini and Parmesan. Season to taste with salt, pepper and dill or nutmeg. Heat, covered, for 2 minutes or until spinach is wilted.

Holiday Fare

We hope the recipes in this special-request chapter help keep your holiday gluten-free!

Lemon Garlic Chicken

SERVES 4

Plan a Greek menu for Easter or any other special occasion. Start with Lemon Garlic Chicken or Souvlaki (see recipe, page 112) with Tzatziki Sauce (see recipe, page 113) and serve with Lemon Jasmine Rice Pilaf (see recipe, page 111) and fresh steamed vegetables.

Tips

Chicken can be marinated at room temperature for up to 30 minutes if you are short of time. Any longer, make sure it is refrigerated. Throw out the plastic bag used for marinating.

Can't find the cover that fits your casserole? Cover it with aluminum foil, dull side out. Trace around the rim with your fingers to be sure foil forms a tight seal.

Substitute an equal amount of oregano for the thyme. Or use 1 tbsp (15 mL) snipped fresh thyme or oregano.

8-cup (2 L) covered casserole dish

1	clove garlic, minced	1
2 tbsp	freshly squeezed lemon juice	25 mL
1 tbsp	extra-virgin olive oil	15 mL
1 tsp	dried thyme	5 mL
¼ tsp	salt	1 mL
Pinch	ground nutmeg	Pinch
Pinch	paprika	Pinch
Pinch	freshly ground white pepper	Pinch
4	skinless boneless chicken breasts	4

1. In a resealable plastic freezer bag set in a bowl, combine garlic, lemon juice, olive oil, thyme, salt, nutmeg, paprika and white pepper. Add chicken breasts to marinade, seal bag and refrigerate for 1 hour.

2. Preheat oven to 375°F (190°C). Place chicken breasts with marinade in the casserole dish, and cover tightly. Bake for 45 minutes, or until juices run clear and meat thermometer registers 170°F (78°C).

Variation

Rather than baking the chicken, barbecue or grill it for 5 to 8 minutes per side.

Lemon Jasmine Rice Pilaf

We are always disappointed when we are served a rice pilaf with only an occasional fleck of vegetable. You don't have to dig for the vegetables in this one, which we like to serve with Lemon Garlic Chicken (see recipe, page 110).

Tips

A pilaf involves frying the rice (or any other grain) in seasonings and herbs to enhance the flavor before cooking liquid is added.

2 to 3 medium-size leeks yield 4 cups (1 L) sliced.

Substitute Vidalia onions for the leeks and GF vegetable stock powder for the chicken stock powder.

Substitute brown, basmati or wild rice, or a combination, for the jasmine rice. Refer to the Rice Cooking Chart on page 14 for cooking times.

1 tbsp	extra-virgin olive oil	15 mL
4 cups	sliced leeks, white and light green parts only	1 L
1 cup	diced carrots	250 mL
1 tsp	dried oregano	5 mL
1 cup	jasmine rice	250 mL
2 cups	water	500 mL
1 tbsp	GF chicken stock powder	15 mL
2 tbsp	grated lemon zest	25 mL
2 tbsp	freshly squeezed lemon juice	25 mL
	Salt and freshly ground white pepper	

1. In a heavy saucepan, heat oil over medium-high heat. Cook leeks, carrots and oregano, stirring occasionally, for 5 to 8 minutes, or until softened. Add rice and cook for 1 minute, stirring constantly.

Stove-Top Method

2. Add water and stock powder and bring to a boil. Reduce heat to low, cover and simmer for 15 minutes, or until rice is tender. Remove saucepan from heat and let stand, covered, for 3 to 5 minutes. Stir in lemon zest and juice and season to taste with salt and pepper. Fluff with a fork.

Microwave Method

2. Transfer rice mixture to a 2 to 3 quart (2 to 3 L) microwaveable casserole dish. Add water and stock powder. Cover and cook on High for 5 minutes, or until boiling. Cook, covered, on Medium (50%), for 15 minutes until liquid is absorbed and rice is tender. Let stand, covered, for 3 to 5 minutes. Stir in lemon zest and juice and season to taste with salt and pepper. Fluff with a fork.

Souvlaki

	SERVES 4	

Everybody loves this traditional Greek dish of marinated lamb chunks cooked on a skewer.

Tips

If desired, prepare the marinade, add the lamb and freeze for up to 1 month. Defrost in the refrigerator for at least 24 hours before cooking.

For faster, more even cooking, leave a space between the meat cubes when threading on the wooden skewers.

Serve over rice or wrapped in 10-inch (25 cm) GF corn tortillas.

Barbecue, grill or broiler, preheated
12-inch (30 cm) wooden skewers

1	clove garlic, coarsely chopped	1
1/3 cup	freshly squeezed lemon juice	75 mL
2 tbsp	extra-virgin olive oil	25 mL
1 tbsp	dried oregano	15 mL
1 tbsp	chopped fresh rosemary	15 mL
1/4 tsp	freshly ground black pepper	1 mL
1 1/2 lb	boneless shoulder or leg of lamb, trimmed and cut into 1-inch (2.5 cm) cubes	750 g

1. In a resealable plastic freezer bag set in a bowl, combine garlic, lemon juice, olive oil, oregano, rosemary and pepper. Add lamb to marinade, seal bag and refrigerate for at least 4 hours or overnight.
2. Meanwhile, soak wooden skewers in water for 30 minutes. Thread lamb cubes evenly on skewers. Barbecue, turning frequently, for 8 to 10 minutes, or until medium-rare or desired doneness.

Variations

Substitute pork tenderloin or chicken breast for the lamb.

If you're in a hurry, drain marinade and place cubes in an 8-inch (2 L) square baking pan; bake in a 350°F (180°C) oven for 30 minutes, or until meat is tender.

Alternate green pepper and onions with the meat on the skewer before grilling.

Tzatziki Sauce

Serve this traditional sauce with souvlaki, or use as a dip with crudités or crackers.

Tips

No need to peel the English cucumber.

Drain the feta well before breaking it into chunks, or purchase crumbled feta.

Let yogurt drain overnight for a thicker sauce.

1½ cups	plain yogurt	375 mL
¼	English cucumber, grated	¼
3	cloves garlic, minced	3
4 oz	feta cheese, broken into chunks (about ¾ cup/175 mL)	125 g
2 tbsp	freshly squeezed lemon juice	25 mL

1. To a strainer lined with damp cheesecloth set inside a bowl, add yogurt. Refrigerate and let drain for 3 to 4 hours, or until reduced by half.
2. To a separate strainer lined with damp cheesecloth set inside a bowl, add grated cucumber. Refrigerate and let drain for 3 to 4 hours or overnight.
3. In a small bowl, combine drained yogurt, drained cucumber, garlic, feta cheese and lemon juice. Refrigerate, covered, for up to 3 days.

Variation

Have extra zucchini and dill in your garden? Substitute zucchini for the cucumber and add 1 tbsp (25 mL) chopped fresh dill.

Summery Yogurt Sauce

Here is a somewhat different sauce to serve with souvlaki. It can be made in less time than it takes the meat to cook.

Tip

Use both the green and the white parts of the green onions.

1½ cups	plain yogurt	375 mL
⅓ cup	diced green onions	75 mL
¼ cup	snipped fresh parsley	50 mL
1	tomato, seeded and diced	1

1. In a small bowl, combine yogurt, green onion, parsley and tomato. Refrigerate, covered, for at least 30 minutes, or until ready to serve. Store in the refrigerator for up to 1 week.

Variation

For a thicker sauce, put yogurt in a strainer lined with damp cheesecloth set inside a bowl, and let it drain overnight in the refrigerator.

Hot Cross Buns

Before its significance for Christians, the cross symbolized the four quarters of the lunar cycle. So ancient Aztecs, Egyptians and Saxons all enjoyed hot cross buns. They have been served on Easter since the early days of the Church.

Tips

In Canada, check for gluten-free confectioner's (icing) sugar. It may contain up to 5% starch, which could be from wheat.

Use a pastry bag and tip to pipe on the icing.

To ensure success, check out the extra information on baking yeast breads on page 67.

Replace the milk in the icing with thawed frozen orange juice concentrate.

To make these lactose-free, replace the milk with water in both the buns and the icing.

Baking sheet, lightly greased

¾ cup	sorghum flour	175 mL
½ cup	whole bean flour	125 mL
⅓ cup	potato starch	75 mL
¼ cup	tapioca starch	50 mL
1 tbsp	xanthan gum	15 mL
2 tsp	bread machine or instant yeast	10 mL
1 tsp	salt	5 mL
1¼ tsp	ground cinnamon	6 mL
¼ tsp	ground cloves	1 mL
¼ tsp	ground nutmeg	1 mL
¾ cup	milk	175 mL
⅓ cup	liquid honey	75 mL
2 tbsp	vegetable oil	25 mL
1 tbsp	fancy molasses	15 mL
1 tsp	cider vinegar	5 mL
2	eggs	2
1 cup	raisins	250 mL

ICING

¾ cup	GF sifted confectioner's (icing) sugar (see tip, at left)	175 mL
1 tbsp	milk	15 mL
¼ tsp	almond extract	1 mL

Bread Machine Method

1. In a large bowl or plastic bag, combine sorghum flour, whole bean flour, potato starch, tapioca starch, xanthan gum, yeast, salt, cinnamon, cloves and nutmeg. Mix well and set aside.

2. Pour milk, honey, oil, molasses and vinegar into the bread machine baking pan. Add eggs.

3. Select the **Dough Cycle**. Allow the liquids to mix until combined. Gradually add the dry ingredients as the bread machine is mixing, scraping sides with a rubber spatula. Incorporate all the dry ingredients within 1 to 2 minutes. Add raisins. Allow the bread machine to complete the cycle.

Mixer Method

1. In a large bowl or plastic bag, combine sorghum flour, whole bean flour, potato starch, tapioca starch, xanthan gum, yeast, salt, cinnamon, cloves and nutmeg. Mix well and set aside.

2. In a separate bowl, using a heavy-duty electric mixer with paddle attachment, combine milk, oil, vinegar and eggs until well blended. Add honey and molasses while mixing.

3. With the mixer on its lowest speed, slowly add the dry ingredients until combined. With a rubber spatula, scrape the bottom and sides of the bowl. With the mixer on medium speed, beat for 4 minutes. Stir in raisins.

For Both Methods

4. Drop batter by heaping spoonfuls onto prepared baking sheet. Using the handle of a wooden spoon or a rubber spatula, make two indents $1/8$ inch (3 cm) deep in the shape of a cross on the top of each bun. Let rise, uncovered, in a warm, draft-free place for 60 to 75 minutes, or until the buns have almost doubled in volume. Meanwhile, preheat oven to 350°F (180°C).

5. Bake for 20 to 25 minutes, or until buns are golden brown. Remove to a cooling rack immediately.

6. *Prepare the icing:* In a small bowl, combine confectioner's sugar, milk and almond extract. Drizzle the crosses of warm buns with icing.

Variation

To prepare California-style buns, add mixed candied peel and dates.

Cornish Game Hens with Cranberry and Wild Rice Stuffing

Susan Hodges, a listserv member, told us about her holiday tradition of serving a "personal turkey" (a.k.a. a Rock Cornish game hen) to her celiac daughter. Here is a stuffing you can use with either "personal" or "family" turkeys.

Tips

Use either a homemade GF chicken stock or a commercial GF chicken stock powder.

When purchasing dried sage or thyme, use dried leaves and avoid the powdered variety.

This recipe makes enough stuffing for a 10-lb (4.5 kg) turkey or for 4 to 6 Cornish game hens.

Roasting pan

4 cups	GF chicken stock	1 L
¾ cup	brown rice	175 mL
½ cup	wild rice, rinsed	125 mL
1 tbsp	crumbled dried sage	15 mL
1 tbsp	crumbled dried thyme	15 mL
1 tbsp	butter	15 mL
1 tbsp	vegetable oil	15 mL
1	large onion, chopped	1
1 cup	sliced cremini mushroom caps (halved then sliced into ¼-inch/0.5 cm pieces)	250 mL
1 cup	diced celery	250 mL
1 cup	diced carrots	250 mL
¼ tsp	salt	1 mL
¼ tsp	freshly ground black pepper	1 mL
1 cup	dried cranberries	250 mL
2 tbsp	balsamic vinegar	25 mL
4 to 6	Cornish game hens (each about 1 to 1¼ lb/500 to 625 g)	4 to 6
	Plum Dipping Sauce (see recipe, page 46)	

1. In a large saucepan, over high heat, combine chicken stock, brown rice, wild rice, sage and thyme and bring to a boil. Reduce heat, cover and simmer gently for 45 to 55 minutes, or until rice is tender. Remove from heat and fluff with a fork. Set aside to cool completely.

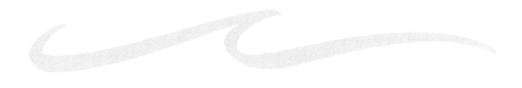

To roast an unstuffed Cornish game hen: Roast uncovered, breast side up, in a preheated 425°F (220°C) oven for 45 minutes. Cut in half before serving.

To bake stuffing outside the hens: Place stuffing in a 3-quart (3 L) casserole dish and stir in ½ cup (125 mL) GF chicken stock. Cover and bake beside the hens.

2. In a skillet, heat butter and oil over medium-high heat. Add onion, mushrooms, celery, carrots, salt and pepper and cook, stirring constantly, until tender, about 8 to 10 minutes. Stir in dried cranberries and balsamic vinegar.

3. Add vegetable mixture to rice mixture and stir gently to combine. Loosely stuff into the game hens and place them breast side up in roasting pan.

4. Preheat oven to 350°F (180°C). Roast hens, uncovered, for 45 to 60 minutes, or until meat thermometer inserted in thigh registers 180°F (82°C). Remove the stuffing immediately.

5. Serve with Plum Dipping Sauce.

Poultry Stuffing Bread
(Bread Machine Method)

The flavor of the herbs bakes right into each bite of this loaf. It's perfect to use in stuffing for Cornish game hens or turkey (see Poultry Stuffing, page 120).

Tips

To ensure success, see page 67 for extra information on baking yeast bread in a bread machine.

Water at 130°F (55°C) will feel hot to the touch.

This is an excellent loaf for making croutons and bread crumbs (see Techniques Glossary, page 179).

Substitute snipped fresh herbs for the dried — you'll need triple the amount. See Techniques Glossary, page 180, for information about working with fresh herbs.

1 1/2 cups	sorghum flour	375 mL
3/4 cup	brown rice flour	175 mL
1/2 cup	potato starch	125 mL
1/4 cup	tapioca starch	50 mL
2 tbsp	granulated sugar	25 mL
1 tbsp	xanthan gum	15 mL
2 tsp	bread machine or instant yeast	10 mL
1 1/2 tsp	salt	7 mL
1/4 cup	snipped fresh parsley	50 mL
3 tbsp	minced dried onion	45 mL
3 tbsp	dried rubbed sage	45 mL
3 tbsp	dried savory	45 mL
1 1/2 tsp	celery seeds	7 mL
1 1/4 cups	water, warmed to 130°F (55°C)	300 mL
1/3 cup	vegetable oil	75 mL
1 tsp	cider vinegar	5 mL
2	eggs	2

1. In a large bowl or plastic bag, combine sorghum flour, brown rice flour, potato starch, tapioca starch, sugar, xanthan gum, yeast, salt, parsley, dried onion, sage, savory and celery seeds. Mix well and set aside.
2. Pour water, oil and vinegar into the bread machine baking pan. Add eggs.
3. Select the **Rapid Two-Hour Basic Cycle.** Allow the liquids to mix until combined. Gradually add the dry ingredients as the bread machine is mixing, scraping sides with a rubber spatula. Incorporate all the dry ingredients within 1 to 2 minutes. Allow the bread machine to complete the cycle. Remove loaf from the pan immediately and let cool completely on a rack.

Poultry Stuffing Bread
(Mixer Method)

MAKES 1 LOAF

The flavor of the herbs bakes right into each bite of this loaf. It's perfect to use in stuffing for Cornish game hens or turkey (see Poultry Stuffing, page 120).

Tips

To ensure success, see page 67 for extra information on baking yeast bread using the mixer method.

This is an excellent loaf for making croutons and bread crumbs (see Techniques Glossary, page 179).

Substitute snipped fresh herbs for the dried — you'll need triple the amount. See Techniques Glossary, page 180, for information about working with fresh herbs.

9- by 5-inch (2 L) loaf pan, lightly greased

1¼ cups	sorghum flour	300 mL
½ cup	brown rice flour	125 mL
⅓ cup	potato starch	75 mL
⅓ cup	tapioca starch	75 mL
1 tbsp	granulated sugar	15 mL
2½ tsp	xanthan gum	12 mL
2 tsp	bread machine or instant yeast	10 mL
1¼ tsp	salt	7 mL
¼ cup	snipped fresh parsley	50 mL
2 tbsp	minced dried onion	25 mL
2 tbsp	dried rubbed sage	25 mL
2 tbsp	dried savory	25 mL
1½ tsp	celery seeds	7 mL
2	eggs	2
1¼ cups	water	300 mL
¼ cup	vegetable oil	50 mL
1 tsp	cider vinegar	5 mL

1. In a large bowl or plastic bag, combine sorghum flour, brown rice flour, potato starch, tapioca starch, sugar, xanthan gum, yeast, salt, parsley, dried onion, sage, savory and celery seeds. Mix well and set aside.

2. In a separate bowl, using a heavy-duty electric mixer with paddle attachment, combine eggs, water, oil and vinegar until well blended.

3. With the mixer on its lowest speed, slowly add the dry ingredients until combined. With a rubber spatula, scrape the bottom and sides of the bowl. With the mixer on medium speed, beat for 4 minutes.

4. Spoon into prepared pan, smoothing top. Let rise, uncovered, in a warm, draft-free place for 60 to 75 minutes, or until dough has risen to the top of the pan. Meanwhile, preheat oven to 350°F (180°C).

5. Bake for 30 to 40 minutes, or until loaf sounds hollow when tapped on the bottom. Remove from the pan immediately and let cool completely on a rack.

Poultry Stuffing

Traditional flavor with a modern twist! We introduced the idea of making stuffing that begins with poultry-seasoned bread crumbs when we first started developing bread machine recipes.

Tips

The United States Department of Agriculture (USDA) and Agriculture Canada both recommend baking stuffing separately, not inside the bird.

Allow 1 cup (250 mL) of stuffing for each 1 lb (500 g) raw poultry.

1	loaf Poultry Stuffing Bread (see recipe, pages 118–19), torn in chunks	1
2 cups	chopped celery	500 mL
1 cup	chopped onions	250 mL

1. In a food processor fitted with a metal blade, pulse bread into coarse crumbs.
2. In a large bowl, combine crumbs, celery and onions.

Baking Stuffing Outside the Bird
3. Place stuffing in a 4-quart (4 L) casserole dish and stir in 1/2 cup (125 mL) pan juices or GF chicken stock. Cover and bake beside the bird for the last hour of roasting.

Baking Stuffing Inside the Bird
3. If you do stuff the bird, loosely fill the cavity and immediately put bird in the oven to roast. Remove the stuffing as soon as the bird is done. Refrigerate leftovers immediately.

Variation

If you want softer, moister stuffing, add 1/2 cup (125 mL) water or GF chicken stock in Step 2.

Turkey Gravy

**MAKES 3 TO 4 CUPS
(750 mL TO 1 L)**

*Crave a hot turkey
sandwich? Be sure to
make extra gravy for
the next day!*

Tips

4 cups (1 L) gravy
is enough for a 15-lb
(6.75 kg) turkey. Recipe
can be doubled or tripled,
but cooking time will
need to be increased
somewhat in each step.

Gravy thickens upon
standing. When
reheating, add extra
liquid a little at a time
until gravy reaches the
desired consistency.
Gravy can be reheated
either on Medium (50%)
in the microwave, or by
simmering over medium-
low heat on the stovetop.

When making gravy and
sauces, substitute an equal
amount of amaranth flour
for the sorghum flour.
This substitution cannot
be made when preparing
cakes, cookies, breads
or pastry.

½ cup	turkey pan drippings	125 mL
½ cup	sorghum flour	125 mL
3 to 4 cups	water, vegetable water or GF chicken stock	750 mL to 1 L
	Salt and freshly ground black pepper	

1. When turkey is removed from the roasting pan, skim fat from juices in pan. Place the pan on the stovetop burners over medium heat or transfer to a saucepan, making sure to scrape all the brown bits. Sprinkle sorghum flour over juices. Cook, stirring constantly, for 1 minute, or until gravy is the consistency of dry sand.

2. Pour in water. Bring to a boil, stirring and scraping up any brown bits from bottom of pan. Reduce heat and simmer, stirring frequently, for 3 to 5 minutes, or until thickened. Add more liquid if necessary. Season to taste with salt and pepper.

Variation

Follow the same method to make beef, pork or chicken gravy.

Carol's Fruit Cake

<table>
<tr><td>MAKES 12 POUNDS
(5.5 KG) ABOUT
21 CUPS (5.25 L)</td></tr>
</table>

Don't halve Carol Coulter's fruitcake recipe — you can begin to enjoy this fruitcake the minute it cools. If you nibble daily, there won't be any left for Christmas. Carol fine-tuned and standardized her recipe in early June to meet our deadline. She measured pans, weighed and measured ingredients, raw batter and the baked cakes, and mailed us a sample. Thanks, Carol — we really appreciate it!

Purchasing Tips

2 cups (500 mL) glacé cherries, citron or mixed peel weigh about 1 lb (500 g).

3 cups (750 mL) seedless golden raisins or Thompson raisins weigh about 1 lb (500 g).

2 cups (500 mL) flat seeded raisins (Muscat, Lexia) weigh about 1 lb (500 g).

2 cups (500 mL) currants weigh about 8 oz (250 g).

Preheat oven to 275°F (140°C)
Two 9- by 5-inch (2 L) loaf pans
Three 7½- by 3½-inch (1 L) loaf pans

2 cups	soy flour	500 mL
1½ cups	tapioca starch	375 mL
½ cup	cornstarch	125 mL
1½ tsp	xanthan gum	7 mL
½ tsp	baking soda	2 mL
½ tsp	salt	2 mL
2 tsp	ground cinnamon	10 mL
1½ tsp	ground nutmeg	7 mL
1 tsp	ground cloves	5 mL
2 lbs	flat seeded raisins (Lexia or Muscat)	1 kg
1 lb	dark seeded raisins (Thompson)	500 g
1 lb	seedless golden raisins	500 g
1 lb	green and red glacé cherries, halved	500 g
1 lb	mixed candied peel	500 g
½ lb	dried currants	250 g
1 cup	butter, softened	250 mL
2 cups	granulated sugar	500 mL
2 cups	packed brown sugar	500 mL
10	eggs	10
1	can (19 oz/540 mL) crushed pineapple, including juice	1
1 tsp	vanilla	5 mL

1. Prepare loaf pans by greasing and completely lining bottoms and sides with a double thickness of heavy brown paper or parchment paper.
2. In a large bowl or plastic bag, mix together soy flour, tapioca starch, cornstarch, xanthan gum, baking soda, salt, cinnamon, nutmeg and cloves; set aside.
3. In a very large bowl or plastic bag, mix together flat, dark and golden raisins, cherries, peel and currants; set aside.

If you don't have a bowl or pot large enough for the whole recipe, use your roasting pan or divide the batter in half before stirring in dried fruit.

Each 9- by 5-inch (2 L) loaf pan holds 5 cups (1.25 L) batter. Each $7^1/_2$- by $3^1/_2$-inch (1 L) loaf pan holds $3^1/_2$ cups (875 mL) batter.

Purchase Muscat or Lexia flat seeded raisins — they are the only varieties with the deep, moist flavor characteristic of a dark fruitcake.

The recipe *can* be halved, if desired.

4. In another very large bowl, using an electric mixer, cream butter, sugar and brown sugar until light and fluffy. Add eggs, one at a time, beating well after each addition; stir in crushed pineapple and vanilla. Gradually beat in dry ingredients, mixing just until smooth. Stir in dried fruit mixture.

5. Spoon into prepared loaf pans, filling only three quarters full; spread to edges and smooth tops with a moist rubber spatula.

6. Position the oven racks to divide the oven into thirds. Fill a large pan with 1 inch (2.5 cm) hot water and place on the bottom shelf.

7. Bake the cakes on the top shelf of preheated oven for about $2^1/_2$ hours for the smaller loaves and about $2^3/_4$ hours for the larger, or until cake tester inserted in the center right to the bottom of the pan comes out without any batter on it. There may be a little sticky raisin or cherry attached to it. Do not overbake.

8. Let cakes cool in the pan on a rack for 10 minutes. Remove cakes from pans to cooling rack. Let cool for 30 minutes before carefully peeling off the paper. Let cool completely before wrapping airtight.

9. Store in the refrigerator for up to 2 months and slice cold from the refrigerator. Or freeze for up to 1 year.

Variations

Add $1^3/_4$ cups (425 mL) whole blanched almonds (about 8 oz/250 g) and 1 cup (250 mL) slivered blanched almonds (about 4 oz/125 g), or $2^3/_4$ cups (675 mL) of chopped walnuts or pecans.

Top the cooled cakes with a thick layer of GF marzipan.

Cranberry Butter Tart Squares

MAKES 3 DOZEN

Barbara Wahn, a local celiac, shared the base recipe with us. She was "determined to make a suitable base to have lots of squares for Christmas." This is the result of several attempts. See page 132 for Coconut Lemon Squares, another recipe that uses Barbara's base.

Tips

Double the recipe and bake in a 13- by 9-inch (3 L) baking pan for 30 to 35 minutes.

Make ahead and freeze in an airtight container for up to 1 month.

See Techniques Glossary, page 179, for information on melting chocolate.

No food processor? Use a pastry blender or two knives to cut the butter into the dry ingredients until mixture resembles small peas. Add the egg and mix until it forms a soft dough.

Preheat oven to 350°F (180°C)
9-inch (2.5 L) square baking pan, lightly greased

BASE

¼ cup	rice flour	50 mL
¾ cup	potato starch	175 mL
3 tbsp	tapioca starch	45 mL
¼ cup	packed brown sugar	50 mL
1 tsp	xanthan gum	5 mL
Pinch	salt	Pinch
½ cup	cold butter, cubed	125 mL
1	egg	1

TOPPING

¾ cup	packed brown sugar	175 mL
1 tbsp	sorghum flour or potato starch	15 mL
¼ tsp	GF baking powder	1 mL
2 tbsp	butter, softened	25 mL
2	eggs, beaten	2
1 tsp	vanilla	5 mL
1 cup	dried cranberries	250 mL
1 cup	raisins	125 mL
½ cup	chopped walnuts	125 mL
1 oz	white chocolate, melted	30 g

1. *Prepare the base:* In a food processor fitted with a metal blade, pulse rice flour, potato starch, tapioca starch, brown sugar, xanthan gum and salt. Add butter and pulse until mixture resembles small peas, about 5 to 10 seconds. With machine running, add egg through feed tube and process until dough just forms a ball. With a moistened rubber or metal spatula, spread evenly in bottom of prepared pan. Bake in preheated oven for 12 to 15 minutes, or until partially set.

2. *Meanwhile, prepare the topping:* In a small bowl or plastic bag, combine brown sugar, sorghum flour and baking powder; set aside. In a medium bowl, using an electric mixer, cream butter, eggs and vanilla. Slowly beat in the dry ingredients until blended. Fold in cranberries, raisins and walnuts.

3. Pour topping over the hot base. Bake for 20 to 25 minutes, or until center is almost firm. Let cool completely in the pan on a cooling rack. Drizzle with melted chocolate and cut into squares.

Variation

Cranberry Pecan Butter Tart Squares: Use an additional 1 cup (250 mL) cranberries instead of the raisins and substitute pecans for the walnuts.

The Bird

Purchasing
- Allow 1 lb (500 g) raw turkey per person. Purchase extra to allow for leftovers.
- For boneless turkey, allow $1/4$ to $1/2$ lb (125 to 250 g) per person.
- Count on 1 cup (250 mL) stuffing for each 1 lb (500 g) of turkey.

Defrosting
- Refrigerator method: Allow $4^1/2$ hours per lb (10 hours per kg).
- Cold water method: Leaving turkey in its original wrapping, cover it with cold water. Change water every hour. Allow 1 hour per lb (2 hours per kg). Cook turkey as soon as it is defrosted.

Roasting
Place turkey, breast side up, on a rack in a large, shallow (no more than $2^1/2$ inches/6 cm deep) roasting pan. Insert a meat thermometer into the thickest part of the thigh, being careful it does not touch the bone. Roast turkey in a preheated 325°F (160°C) oven. See chart below for roasting times, or roast until the thermometer registers 180°F (82°C) in the thigh, 170°F (78°C) in the breast and 165°F (74°C) in the stuffing. (Note: The United States Department of Agriculture (USDA) and Agriculture Canada both recommend baking stuffing separately, not inside the bird.) Remove turkey from the oven and allow the bird to rest, tented loosely with foil, for 15 to 20 minutes before carving.

ROASTING TIMES FOR TURKEY*

Weight	Stuffed	Unstuffed
6 to 8 lbs (3 to 3.5 kg)	3 to $3^1/4$ hours	$2^1/2$ to $2^3/4$ hours
8 to 10 lbs (3.5 to 4.5 kg)	$3^1/4$ to $3^1/2$ hours	$2^3/4$ to 3 hours
10 to 12 lbs (4.5 to 5.5 kg)	$3^1/2$ to $3^3/4$ hours	3 to $3^1/4$ hours
12 to 16 lbs (5.5 to 7 kg)	$3^3/4$ to 4 hours	$3^1/4$ to $3^1/2$ hours
16 to 22 lbs (7 to 10 kg)	4 to $4^1/2$ hours	$3^1/2$ to 4 hours

* Canadian Turkey Marketing Agency

Leftovers
- Refrigerate or freeze leftover turkey within 1 hour of roasting.
- Take the meat off the bones to cool it more quickly. Store leftover turkey in the refrigerator for 4 to 6 days or in the freezer for 4 to 6 months. Label and date the containers.
- When packaging warm leftovers, use airtight containers no more than 2 to 3 inches (5 to 7.5 cm) deep.
- Place in the coldest part of the refrigerator or freezer with 1 to 2 inches (2 to 5 cm) of space around each container. This promotes quick, even cooling.
- When you reheat leftovers, make sure the internal temperature reaches 165°F (74°C).
- Sauces, soups and gravies should be brought to a rolling boil before serving.

Cookies and Bars

Ideas for your next cookie exchange!

Cranberry Pistachio Biscotti

MAKES 64 COOKIES

These have the appearance and texture of traditional twice-baked biscotti, but are much easier and faster to make. We like to dip them in a sweet Italian dessert wine, or in coffee.

Tips

Biscotti will be medium-firm and crunchy; for softer biscotti, bake for only 10 minutes in Step 5; for very firm biscotti, bake for 20 minutes.

Store in an airtight container at room temperature for up to 3 weeks, or freeze for up to 2 months.

If you prefer, you can use a 13- by 9-inch (3 L) baking pan instead of the two 8-inch (2 L) pans.

Try orange-flavored cranberries and substitute orange zest for the lemon zest.

Substitute pecans or hazelnuts for the pistachios.

Preheat oven to 325°F (160°C)
Two 8-inch (2 L) square baking pans, foil-lined and lightly greased
Baking sheets, ungreased

1½ cups	amaranth flour	375 mL
½ cup	soy flour	125 mL
⅓ cup	potato starch	75 mL
¼ cup	tapioca starch	50 mL
1½ tsp	xanthan gum	7 mL
1 tsp	GF baking powder	5 mL
Pinch	salt	Pinch
4	eggs	4
1¼ cups	granulated sugar	300 mL
1 tbsp	grated lemon zest	15 mL
1 tsp	vanilla	5 mL
1½ cups	coarsely chopped pistachios	375 mL
1 cup	dried cranberries	250 mL

1. In a large bowl or plastic bag, combine amaranth flour, soy flour, potato starch, tapioca starch, xanthan gum, baking powder and salt. Mix well and set aside.

2. In a separate bowl, using an electric mixer, beat eggs, sugar, lemon zest and vanilla until combined.

3. Slowly beat in dry ingredients and mix just until combined. Stir in pistachios and cranberries. Spoon into prepared pans. Using a moistened rubber spatula, spread batter to edges and smooth tops.

4. Bake in preheated oven for 30 to 35 minutes, or until firm or tops are just turning golden. Let cool in pans for 5 minutes.

5. Remove from pans, remove foil and let cool on a cutting board for 5 minutes. Cut into quarters, then cut each quarter into 8 slices. Arrange slices upright (cut sides exposed) at least ½ inch (1 cm) apart on baking sheets. Bake for an additional 15 minutes, until dry and crisp. Transfer to a cooling rack immediately.

Poultry Stuffing (page 120)

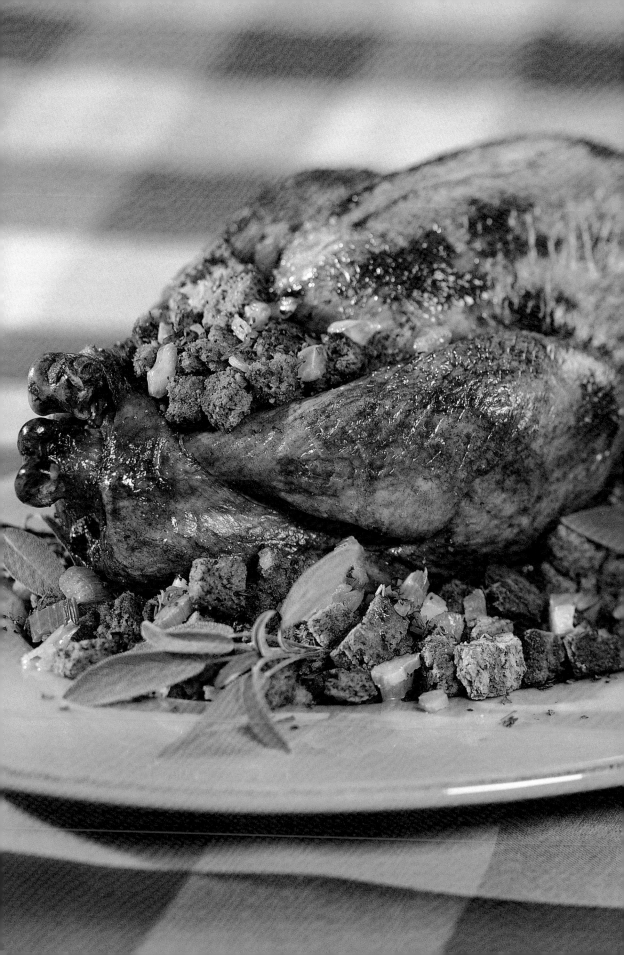

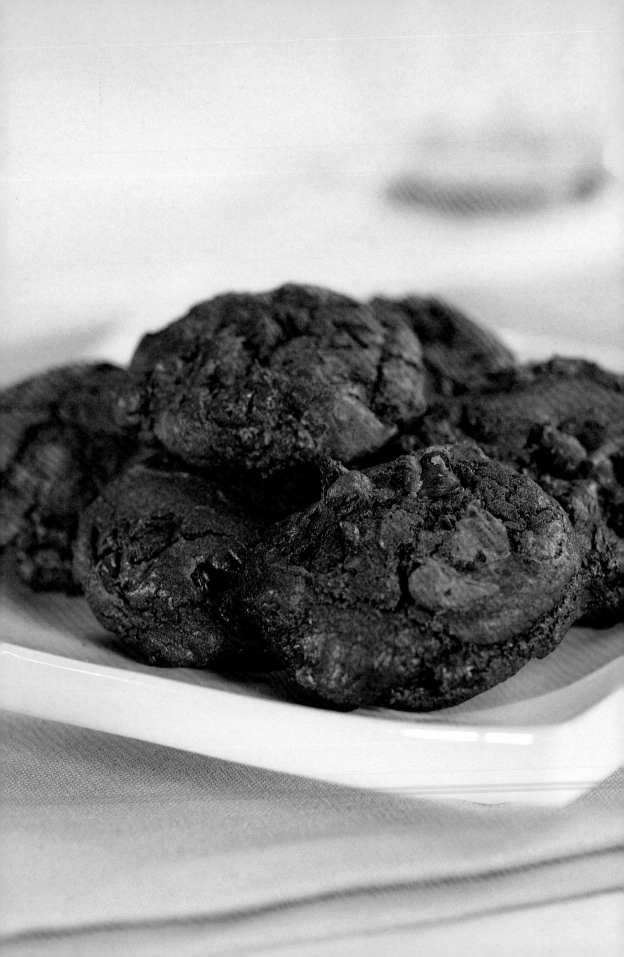

Crunchy Flaxseed Cookies

These perfect back-to-school lunchbox treats will remind you of oatmeal cookies. We dare you to eat just one!

Tips

We tried this cookie with sprouted flax powder, flax meal, ground flaxseed and flax flour. All were delicious, so you can substitute one for another.

Whole flaxseed can be stored at room temperature for up to 1 year. Ground flaxseed can be stored in the refrigerator for up to 90 days, but for optimum freshness it is best to grind it as you need it.

This dough doesn't hold in the refrigerator or freezer. We tried to make these into refrigerator slice-and-bake cookies — we don't recommend it.

Substitute raw hemp powder for ground flaxseed and hemp hearts® for half the cracked flaxseed.

Preheat oven to 350°F (180°C)
Baking sheets, lightly greased

⅓ cup	sorghum flour	75 mL
¼ cup	whole bean flour	50 mL
¼ cup	tapioca starch	50 mL
¼ cup	ground flaxseed	50 mL
⅔ cup	cracked flaxseed	150 mL
1 tsp	baking soda	5 mL
1 tsp	xanthan gum	5 mL
¼ tsp	salt	1 mL
½ cup	butter or shortening, softened	125 mL
½ cup	packed brown sugar	125 mL
⅓ cup	granulated sugar	75 mL
1	egg	1
½ tsp	vanilla	2 mL
⅔ cup	buckwheat flakes	150 mL

1. In a medium bowl or plastic bag, combine sorghum flour, whole bean flour, tapioca starch, ground flaxseed, cracked flaxseed, baking soda, xanthan gum and salt. Mix well and set aside.

2. In a large bowl, using an electric mixer, cream the butter, brown sugar and granulated sugar until combined. Add egg and vanilla and cream until light and fluffy. Slowly beat in the dry ingredients until combined. Stir in buckwheat flakes. Roll into 1-inch (2.5 cm) balls. Place 2 inches (5 cm) apart on prepared baking sheets and flatten with a fork or the bottom of a drinking glass.

3. Bake in preheated oven for 10 to 15 minutes, or until set. Remove from baking sheets to cooling rack immediately.

Variation

Make date- or jam-filled sandwich cookies or add 1 cup (250 mL) chocolate chips or raisins to the batter and bake as drop cookies.

Triple-Threat Mocha Chocolate Chip Cookies (page 131)

Molasses Cookies

Hermit-like in color and flavor — an excellent cookie for packed lunches.

Tips

Keep a close eye on the oven, as these cookies burn easily.

Cookies spread and are still soft when baked; if baked too long, cookies become very crunchy when cold.

Make ahead and freeze for up to 2 months in an airtight container.

Substitute whole bean flour, yellow or green pea flour or garbanzo-fava (garfava) bean flour for the chickpea flour.

Baking sheets, lightly greased

1²/₃ cups	sorghum flour	400 mL
1 cup	chickpea (garbanzo bean) flour	250 mL
1/₃ cup	tapioca starch	75 mL
1 tsp	baking soda	5 mL
1 tsp	xanthan gum	5 mL
1/₂ tsp	salt	2 mL
1 tsp	ground cinnamon	5 mL
1/₂ tsp	ground allspice	2 mL
1/₂ tsp	ground cloves	2 mL
1 cup	shortening or butter, softened	250 mL
2	eggs	2
1 cup	fancy molasses	250 mL
3/₄ cup	granulated sugar	175 mL
2 tbsp	Orange Marmalade (see recipe, page 90)	25 mL
2 cups	raisins	500 mL
2 cups	chopped walnuts	500 mL

1. In a large bowl or plastic bag, combine sorghum flour, chickpea flour, tapioca starch, baking soda, xanthan gum, salt, cinnamon, allspice and cloves. Mix well and set aside.

2. In another large bowl, using an electric mixer, cream shortening, eggs, molasses, sugar and marmalade. Slowly beat in the dry ingredients until combined. Stir in raisins and walnuts. Drop dough by rounded spoonfuls 2 inches (5 cm) apart on prepared baking sheets. Let stand for 30 minutes. Meanwhile, preheat oven to 350°F (180°C).

3. Bake in preheated oven for 10 to 12 minutes, or until set. Transfer to a cooling rack immediately.

Triple-Threat Mocha Chocolate Chip Cookies

Triple the pleasure, triple the fun — but who's counting calories? These fudgy morsels are worth every bite!

Tips

Cookies spread and are still soft when baked; if baked too long, cookies become very crunchy when cold.

For crisper cookies, use ²/₃ cup (150 mL) butter instead of half butter and half shortening.

Make ahead and freeze for up to 2 months in an airtight container.

Substitute chickpea (garbanzo bean) flour, yellow or green pea flour or garbanzo-fava (garfava) bean flour for the whole bean flour.

Baking sheets, lightly greased

1 cup	sorghum flour	250 mL
²/₃ cup	whole bean flour	150 mL
¹/₂ cup	tapioca starch	125 mL
1 tsp	baking soda	5 mL
1 tsp	xanthan gum	5 mL
¹/₂ tsp	salt	2 mL
¹/₃ cup	unsweetened cocoa powder, sifted	75 mL
4 oz	semi-sweet chocolate	125 g
¹/₃ cup	butter	75 mL
¹/₃ cup	shortening	75 mL
2 tbsp	water	25 mL
1 tbsp	instant coffee granules	15 mL
2	eggs	2
²/₃ cup	granulated sugar	150 mL
²/₃ cup	packed brown sugar	150 mL
1¹/₂ tsp	vanilla	7 mL
1 cup	semi-sweet chocolate chips	250 mL

1. In a large bowl or plastic bag, combine sorghum flour, whole bean flour, tapioca starch, baking soda, xanthan gum, salt and cocoa. Mix well and set aside.

2. In a medium microwave-safe bowl, microwave chocolate, butter, shortening, water and coffee granules, uncovered, on Medium (50 %) for 2 minutes. Stir until completely melted. Set aside to cool.

3. In a large bowl, using an electric mixer, beat eggs, sugar and brown sugar for 3 minutes, until smooth. Add vanilla and cooled melted chocolate mixture. Slowly beat in the dry ingredients until combined. Stir in chocolate chips. Drop dough by rounded spoonfuls 2 inches (5 cm) apart on prepared baking sheets. Let stand for 30 minutes. Meanwhile, preheat oven to 350°F (180°C).

4. Bake in preheated oven for 10 to 12 minutes, or until set. Transfer to a cooling rack immediately.

Coconut Lemon Squares

MAKES 3 DOZEN SQUARES

Try our delicious simplified version of lemony three-layer squares. The coconut rises to the top during baking to finish the squares with a crisp topping.

Tips

The zest and juice of the fresh lemon enhances the flavor. To get more juice out of it, roll the lemon, brought to room temperature, on the counter or between your hands.

No food processor? Use a pastry blender or two knives to cut the butter into the dry ingredients until the mixture resembles small peas. Add the egg and mix until it forms a soft dough.

Double the recipe and bake in a 13- by 9-inch (3 L) baking pan. Baking time may need to be increased by 5 to 10 minutes.

Preheat oven to 350°F (180°C)
9-inch (2.5 L) square baking pan, lightly greased and lined with parchment paper

BASE

¼ cup	rice flour	50 mL
¾ cup	cornstarch	175 mL
3 tbsp	tapioca starch	45 mL
1 tsp	xanthan gum	5 mL
¼ cup	packed brown sugar	50 mL
Pinch	salt	Pinch
½ cup	unsweetened shredded coconut	125 mL
½ cup	cold butter, cubed	125 mL
1	egg	1

TOPPING

4	eggs	4
1½ cups	granulated sugar	375 mL
1 cup	unsweetened shredded coconut	250 mL
2 tbsp	grated lemon zest	25 mL
½ cup	freshly squeezed lemon juice	125 mL
¼ cup	cornstarch	50 mL
1 tsp	GF baking powder	5 mL

1. *Prepare the base:* In a food processor fitted with a metal blade, pulse rice flour, cornstarch, tapioca starch, xanthan gum, brown sugar, salt and coconut. Add butter and pulse until mixture resembles small peas, about 5 to 10 seconds. With machine running, add egg through feed tube. Process until dough just forms a ball. Spread evenly in bottom of prepared pan. Using a moistened rubber or metal spatula, spread to edges and smooth top . Remoisten when dough begins to stick to spatula.

2. Bake in preheated oven for 12 to 15 minutes, or until set. Reduce oven temperature to 325°F (160°C).

Cool squares completely before cutting. To prevent tearing, dip a sharp knife in hot water and wipe with a cloth after each cut.

Make ahead and freeze in an airtight container for up to 2 weeks.

3. *Meanwhile, prepare the topping:* In a bowl, using an electric mixer, beat together eggs, sugar, coconut, lemon zest, lemon juice, cornstarch and baking powder until blended. Pour over the hot base.
4. Bake for 40 to 45 minutes, or until lightly browned and firm to the touch. Let cool completely in the pan on a rack. Cut into squares.

Variation

To turn these into lemon squares, omit the coconut from both the base and the topping.

Cookies Through the Mail

Everyone appreciates receiving a "care package" from home. Here are some tips to help you get it there intact:

1. Select recipes for soft, chewy cookies: they are less likely to crumble. Those baked with sorghum flour travel better than those baked with rice flour.
2. Slice refrigerator cookie dough a bit thicker than usual to avoid breakage.
3. Squares are easier to pack than cookies.
4. Wrap cookies individually or in pairs, with two bottoms sandwiched together. Layer individual cookies in potato chip cylinders with a circle of waxed or parchment paper between them.
5. Place wrapped cookies into individual paper muffin liners. Choose colorful liners for holidays and special occasions.
6. Plan to mail parcels on the same day the cookies are baked.
7. Fill boxes to within 1 inch (2.5 cm) of the top and then add crumpled plastic wrap or bubble wrap to cushion the contents.
8. Pack cookies in several small boxes rather than one large one. Then place the smaller boxes inside a larger box and cushion them with Styrofoam packing peanuts. Seal tightly and mark "fragile."

Pumpkin Date Bars

These quick and easy, lactose-free, moist bars are dotted with dates, nuts and a refreshing touch of orange. No need to frost; simply dust with GF confectioner's (icing) sugar, if desired.

Tips

Check for gluten-free confectioner's (icing) sugar. In Canada, it may contain up to 5% starch, which could be from wheat.

Store in an airtight container at room temperature for up to 5 days or freeze for up to 2 months.

Substitute an equal amount of dried cranberries for the walnuts.

For a stronger orange flavor, add 1/2 tsp (2 mL) orange extract.

9-inch (2.5 L) square baking pan, lined with foil, lightly greased

3/4 cup	soy flour	175 mL
1/2 cup	packed brown sugar	125 mL
1 1/2 tsp	xanthan gum	7 mL
2 tsp	GF baking powder	10 mL
1/2 tsp	salt	2 mL
2 tbsp	grated orange zest	25 mL
1/2 tsp	ground cinnamon	2 mL
1/2 tsp	ground nutmeg	2 mL
2	eggs	2
1/2 cup	canned pumpkin purée (not pie filling)	125 mL
2 tbsp	vegetable oil	25 mL
3/4 cup	chopped pitted dates	175 mL
1/2 cup	chopped walnuts	125 mL

1. In a large bowl or plastic bag, mix together soy flour, brown sugar, xanthan gum, baking powder, salt, orange zest, cinnamon and nutmeg. Set aside.

2. In another large bowl, using an electric mixer, beat eggs, pumpkin purée and oil until combined. Slowly beat in the dry ingredients and mix just until combined. Stir in dates and walnuts. Spoon into prepared pan. Using a moistened rubber spatula, spread to edges and smooth top. Let stand for 30 minutes. Meanwhile, preheat oven to 325°F (160°C).

3. Bake in preheated oven for 25 to 30 minutes, or until a cake tester inserted in the center comes out clean. Let cool completely in the pan on a rack. Cut into small bars.

Chocolate-Coated Peanut Blondies

Blond brownies, or blondies, continue to gain in popularity. Here is a flavor kids of any age will enjoy — perfect for lunches and snacks.

Tips

Spread the melted chocolate chips over the hot blondies with the back of a spoon or a spatula as soon as they come out of the oven.

Don't substitute dry-roasted peanuts, as they may contain gluten.

Substitute GF peanut butter chips for the chocolate chips.

9-inch (2.5 L) square baking pan, lightly greased

¾ cup	soy flour	175 mL
⅓ cup	whole bean flour	75 mL
2 tbsp	tapioca starch	25 mL
1½ tsp	xanthan gum	7 mL
1 tbsp	GF baking powder	15 mL
½ cup	butter or shortening, softened	125 mL
½ cup	GF peanut butter	125 mL
⅔ cup	packed brown sugar	150 mL
3	eggs	3
2 tsp	vanilla	10 mL
1 cup	chopped peanuts	250 mL
1 cup	chocolate chips	250 mL

1. In a small bowl or plastic bag, combine soy flour, whole bean flour, tapioca starch, xanthan gum and baking powder. Mix well and set aside.
2. In a large bowl, using an electric mixer, cream butter, peanut butter and brown sugar until well blended. Add eggs and vanilla and cream until light and fluffy. Slowly beat in the dry ingredients until combined. Stir in peanuts. Spoon into prepared pan. Using a moistened rubber spatula, spread to edges and smooth top. Sprinkle with chocolate chips. Let stand for 30 minutes. Meanwhile, preheat oven to 325°F (160°C).
3. Bake in preheated oven 30 to 35 minutes, or until a wooden skewer inserted in the center comes out clean. Spread melted chocolate chips to evenly cover the top. Let cool completely on a rack. Cut into bars.

Variation

Apricot Almond Blondies: Substitute 1 cup (250 mL) chopped dried apricots and ½ cup (125 mL) toasted slivered almonds for the peanuts and ½ cup (125 mL) apricot jam for the chocolate chips.

Buckwheat Date Squares

MAKES 16 SQUARES
OR 8 DESSERT
SQUARES

We both consider these comfort food — we know you will enjoy them either in smaller squares for snacks or in larger pieces for dessert.

Tips

When purchasing chopped dates, check for wheat starch in the coating.

Recipe can easily be doubled and baked in a 13- by 9-inch (3 L) baking pan for 30 to 40 minutes.

Squares can be stored in an airtight container at room temperature for 5 days or frozen for up to 2 months.

Substitute GF mincemeat or green tomato mincemeat for the date filling. No need to cook the filling first.

Preheat oven to 350°F (180°C)
8-inch (2 L) square baking pan, lightly greased

DATE FILLING

1¼ cups	chopped pitted dates	300 mL
¾ cup	water	175 mL

CRUMB CRUST

½ cup	pea flour	125 mL
¼ cup	pecan flour	50 mL
¾ cup	buckwheat flakes	175 mL
¼ tsp	baking soda	1 mL
¼ tsp	salt	1 mL
1 tsp	ground cinnamon	5 tsp
¼ cup	butter or margarine, softened	50 mL
½ cup	packed brown sugar	125 mL

1. *Prepare the date filling:* In a saucepan, over medium heat, heat dates and water until the mixture comes to a boil. Reduce heat to medium-low, cover and simmer for 6 minutes, stirring frequently, until mixture is the consistency of jam. Set aside.

2. *Prepare the crumb crust:* In a small bowl or plastic bag, combine pea flour, pecan flour, buckwheat flakes, baking soda, salt and cinnamon. Mix well and set aside.

3. In a medium bowl, cream butter and brown sugar. Slowly beat in the dry ingredients. Mix until crumbly. Firmly pat two-thirds of the mixture into prepared pan. Top with date filling and sprinkle with remaining crumb mixture.

4. Bake in preheated oven for 20 to 30 minutes, or until light golden brown. Let cool completely on a rack. Cut into squares.

Rich Cookie Dough

Want to make an assortment of cookies without making dozens of each kind? Start with this basic shortbread-style recipe, divide the dough into portions and make several varieties.

Tips

1 lb (500 g) of butter yields 2 cups (500 mL).

Set butter out on kitchen counter the night before you plan to make this cookie mix.

1 cup	amaranth flour	250 mL
1 cup	GF confectioner's (icing) sugar	250 mL
1⅓ cups	cornstarch	325 mL
4 tsp	xanthan gum	20 mL
1¼ tsp	salt	6 mL
2 cups	butter, softened	500 mL
½ cup	packed brown sugar	125 mL
2	eggs	2

1. In a large bowl or plastic bag, combine amaranth flour, confectioner's sugar, cornstarch, xanthan gum and salt. Set aside.

2. In another large bowl, using an electric mixer, beat butter, brown sugar and eggs just until smooth. Slowly beat in dry ingredients until combined, occasionally scraping the bottom and sides of bowl with a rubber spatula.

3. Divide dough into four portions. For each, select a variation from the recipes on pages 138 to 142.

Additional Tips for Rich Cookie Dough

1. If dough becomes too soft, refrigerate for at least 15 minutes.
2. Roll out the dough to a uniform thickness for more even baking. Cut out shapes as close together as possible. Use as little flour as possible when re-rolling dough. Sweet rice flour works well here.
3. Store dough wrapped airtight in the refrigerator for up to 5 days or freeze for up to 2 months. Thaw in the refrigerator overnight. Bring to room temperature before using.
4. During baking, keep your eyes on the oven, not the clock — 1 to 2 minutes can mean the difference between undercooked and burnt shortbread.
5. When using 2 baking sheets, place them in the upper and lower thirds of the oven. Switch their positions halfway through the baking time.
6. Layer the baked cookies between waxed paper in an airtight container and store at room temperature for up to 5 days or freeze for up to 2 weeks.

Orange Pecan Crescents

When dipped in chocolate, these shortbread-like crescents will be the first to disappear.

Tips

If pecan flour is not readily available in your area, see Techniques Glossary, page 181, under Nut flour, for instructions on making your own.

If batter is slightly sticky, dust your hands with GF confectioner's (icing) sugar or sweet rice flour before shaping each cookie.

Preheat oven to 350°F (180°C)
Baking sheet, lightly greased

¼ batch	Rich Cookie Dough (see recipe, page 137)	¼ batch
⅓ cup	pecan flour	75 mL
¼ cup	amaranth flour	50 mL
½ cup	chopped pecans	125 mL
2 tbsp	grated orange zest	25 mL

1. In a medium bowl, combine Rich Cookie Dough, pecan flour, amaranth flour, pecans and orange zest. Gather the dough into a ball, kneading in any dry ingredients. Shape into logs 2½ inches (6 cm) long and ½ inch (1 cm) thick, then bend into crescents. Place crescents 1 inch (2.5 cm) apart on prepared baking sheet.

2. Bake in preheated oven for 12 to 15 minutes, or until lightly browned. Transfer to a rack and let cool completely.

Variations

Dip one end of completely cooled cookies in melted chocolate. See Techniques Glossary, page 179, for instructions on melting chocolate.

Add ½ cup (125 mL) dried cranberries to the dough.

While still hot from the oven, roll cookies in GF confectioner's (icing) sugar.

Lemon Hazelnut Snowballs

White as snowballs, melt-in-your-mouth goodness!

Tips

If batter is slightly sticky, dust your hands with GF confectioner's (icing) sugar or sweet rice flour before shaping each cookie.

Layer cookies between waxed paper in an airtight container and store at room temperature for up to 1 week or freeze for up to 2 months.

When entertaining, set each cookie in a decorative miniature paper liner.

Preheat oven to 350°F (180°C)
Baking sheet, lightly greased

¼ batch	Rich Cookie Dough (see recipe, page 137)	¼ batch
½ cup	hazelnut flour	125 mL
¼ cup	amaranth flour	50 mL
½ cup	chopped hazelnuts	125 mL
2 tbsp	grated lemon zest	25 mL
	GF confectioner's (icing) sugar	

1. In a medium bowl, combine Rich Cookie Dough, hazelnut flour, amaranth flour, hazelnuts and lemon zest. Gather the dough into a ball, kneading in any dry ingredients. Roll into 1-inch (2.5 cm) balls. Place 1 inch (2.5 cm) apart on prepared baking sheet.

2. Bake in preheated oven for 12 to 15 minutes, or until lightly browned. Transfer to a rack. Let cool for 5 minutes.

3. Sift confectioner's sugar into a small bowl and roll balls in confectioner's sugar. Return to rack and let cool completely. If desired, roll in confectioner's sugar a second time.

Variation

Choose any other cookie shape from this section.

Chocolate Chip Bars

Here's a flavor combination everyone with a sweet tooth will love: chocolate and hazelnuts!

Tips

If batter is slightly sticky, spread with a moistened spatula.

Substitute white chocolate chips or toffee bits for the chocolate chips and macadamia nuts for the hazelnuts.

Preheat oven to 350°F (180°C)
8-inch (2 L) square baking pan, lightly greased

¼ batch	Rich Cookie Dough (see recipe, page 137)	¼ batch
⅓ cup	sorghum flour	75 mL
⅓ cup	whole bean flour	75 mL
¾ cup	chocolate chips	175 mL
½ cup	chopped hazelnuts	125 mL
1 tsp	almond extract	5 mL

1. In a medium bowl, combine Rich Cookie Dough, sorghum flour, bean flour, chocolate chips, hazelnuts and almond extract. Mix well. Press into prepared pan.
2. Bake in preheated oven for 25 to 30 minutes, or until lightly browned. Transfer to a rack. Let cool completely before cutting into bars.

Lemon Poppy Drops

Our friend Tom insisted we include his favorite cookie — a lemon poppy seed recipe.

Tips

You can keep extra freshly squeezed lemon juice and freshly grated lemon zest in the freezer for up to 6 months.

Substitute orange zest and juice for the lemon.

Preheat oven to 350°F (180°C)
Baking sheet, lightly greased

¼ batch	Rich Cookie Dough (see recipe, page 137)	¼ batch
½ cup	amaranth flour	125 mL
2 tbsp	poppy seeds	25 mL
2 tbsp	grated lemon zest	25 mL
2 tbsp	freshly squeezed lemon juice	25 mL

1. In a medium bowl, combine Rich Cookie Dough, amaranth flour, poppy seeds, lemon zest and juice. Drop by heaping tablespoonfuls (15 mL) 1½ inches (4 cm) apart on prepared baking sheet.
2. Bake in preheated oven for 12 to 15 minutes, or until lightly browned. Immediately transfer to a rack and let cool completely.

Crunchy Mocha Cookies

MAKES 2 DOZEN COOKIES

You may think these look like peanut butter cookies, but wait till you taste them!

Tips

The thinner you press the cookies, the crunchier they are when baked.

For a softer cookie, substitute granulated sugar for the brown.

Substitute an equal amount of yellow pea flour for the whole bean flour.

Preheat oven to 350°F (180°C)
Baking sheet, lightly greased

1/3 cup	whole bean flour	75 mL
1/4 cup	sorghum flour	50 mL
1/4 cup	packed brown sugar	50 mL
2 tbsp	unsweetened cocoa powder	25 mL
2 tsp	instant coffee granules	10 mL
1/4 batch	Rich Cookie Dough (see recipe, page 137)	1/4 batch
	Sweet rice flour	

1. In a medium bowl, sift together whole bean flour, sorghum flour, brown sugar, cocoa powder and coffee granules. Add Rich Cookie Dough and combine with a wooden spoon until blended. Roll into 1-inch (2.5 cm) balls. Place 1 1/2 inches (4 cm) apart on prepared baking sheet. Flatten slightly with a fork dipped in sweet rice flour.
2. Bake in preheated oven for 12 to 15 minutes, or until puffed and firm around the edges. Immediately transfer to a rack and let cool completely.

Variations

For coffee-flavored cookies, omit the cocoa.

Roll 1-inch (2.5 cm) balls in finely chopped nuts of your choice.

Parmesan Rosemary Slices

*A savory cracker to go on a
cheese and cracker platter.*

Tips

Logs can be frozen in
an airtight container for
up to 1 month. To bake,
thaw slightly and cut into
slices ⅓ inch (0.7 cm)
thick. Bake for 10 to
12 minutes.

Store baked slices in
an airtight container at
room temperature for
up to 5 days or freeze
for up to 2 months.

Substitute grated
Romano or Asiago
cheese for the Parmesan.

Preheat oven to 350°F (180°C)
Baking sheet, lightly greased

¼ batch	Rich Cookie Dough (see recipe, page 137)	¼ batch
⅓ cup	soy flour	75 mL
⅓ cup	freshly grated Parmesan cheese	75 mL
2 tbsp	chopped fresh rosemary	25 mL

1. In a medium bowl, combine Rich Cookie Dough, soy flour, Parmesan and rosemary. Form into a log 1½ inches (4 cm) in diameter. Wrap in plastic wrap and refrigerate for at least 2 hours, until firm, or for up to 3 days (or freeze for up to 3 weeks).

2. Let stand at room temperature for 20 minutes. Cut log into slices ⅓ inch (0.7 cm) thick. Place 1½ inches (4 cm) apart on prepared baking sheet.

3. Bake in preheated oven for 10 to 12 minutes, or until lightly browned. Immediately transfer to a rack and let cool completely.

Sweet Endings

We all crave sweets to finish off a meal or to enjoy with a hot cup of tea. Don't wait until you're having company to bake these recipes.

Banana Poppy Seed Cake

For those who love their bananas with poppy seeds. The best part is you can eat this delight when you're on the run — the slices are the perfect size to carry with you.

Tips

The batter should fill the pan half-full.

Instead of greasing, line the bottom of the tube pan with parchment or waxed paper. Remove the tube and trace the bottom. Invert and trace the center. Cut the center circle large enough so that the parchment paper slips over the tube.

Substitute any variety of bean flour for the yellow pea flour.

10-inch (4 L) tube or 10-inch (3 L) Bundt pan, lightly greased

1 cup	sorghum flour	250 mL
1/2 cup	yellow pea flour	125 mL
1/4 cup	potato starch	50 mL
1/4 cup	tapioca starch	50 mL
1 1/2 tsp	xanthan gum	7 mL
1 tbsp	GF baking powder	15 mL
1 tsp	baking soda	5 mL
1/4 tsp	salt	1 mL
3 tbsp	poppy seeds	45 mL
1/2 tsp	ground nutmeg	2 mL
2	eggs	2
2 cups	mashed banana	500 mL
1/2 cup	packed brown sugar	125 mL
1/4 cup	vegetable oil	50 mL
1 tsp	cider vinegar	5 mL

1. In a large bowl or plastic bag, combine sorghum flour, pea flour, potato starch, tapioca starch, xanthan gum, baking powder, baking soda, salt, poppy seeds and nutmeg. Mix well and set aside.

2. In another large bowl, using an electric mixer, beat eggs, banana, brown sugar, oil and vinegar until combined. Add dry ingredients and mix just until combined. Spoon batter into prepared pan, Using a moistened rubber spatula, spread to edges and smooth top. Let stand for 30 minutes. Meanwhile, preheat oven to 325°F (160°C).

3. Bake in preheated oven for 40 to 45 minutes, or until a cake tester inserted in the center comes out clean. Let cake cool in the pan on a rack for 10 minutes. Remove from pan and let cool completely on a rack.

Variation

For crunch, add 3/4 cup (175 mL) chopped pecans, walnuts or hazelnuts.

Almond Sponge Cake

SERVES 12 TO 16

The perfect cake — light, airy, and not too sweet! Serve topped with fresh fruit and drizzled with Simple Hot Fudge Sauce (see recipe, page 157).

Tips

This is the ideal time to use liquid egg whites purchased in cartons. Substitute 1¼ cups (300 mL) liquid egg whites for the 10 egg whites.

Make sure the mixer bowl, wire whisk attachment, rubber spatula and tube pan are completely free of grease.

To slice without squishing cake, use dental floss or a knife with a serrated edge, such as an electric knife.

For instructions on making your own almond flour, see Techniques Glossary, page 181, under Nut flour.

For instructions on warming egg whites and yolks to room temperature, see Techniques Glossary, page 179.

Substitute amaranth flour for the almond flour.

Preheat oven to 350°F (180°C)
10-inch (4 L) tube pan, ungreased, bottom lined with parchment paper

½ cup	almond flour	125 mL
⅓ cup	cornstarch	75 mL
1 tsp	xanthan gum	5 mL
10	egg whites, at room temperature	10
1 tbsp	freshly squeezed lemon juice	15 mL
1½ tsp	cream of tartar	7 mL
1 tsp	almond extract	5 mL
¼ tsp	salt	1 mL
⅓ cup	granulated sugar	75 mL
4	egg yolks, at room temperature	4
¼ cup	granulated sugar	50 mL

1. In a small bowl or plastic bag, combine almond flour, cornstarch and xanthan gum. Set aside.

2. In a large bowl, using an electric mixer with wire whisk attachment, beat egg whites until foamy. While beating, add lemon juice, cream of tartar, almond extract and salt. Continue to beat until egg whites form stiff peaks. Gradually add the ⅓ cup (75 mL) sugar. Continue to beat until mixture is very stiff and glossy but not dry.

3. In a small deep bowl, using an electric mixer, beat egg yolks and the ¼ cup (50 mL) sugar until thick and pale-lemon in color, approximately 5 minutes. Fold egg yolks into beaten egg white mixture. Sift in dry ingredients, one-third at a time. Gently fold in each addition until well blended. Spoon into prepared pan.

4. Bake in preheated oven for 25 to 30 minutes, or until cake is golden and springs back when lightly touched. Invert pan over a funnel or bottle until completely cooled. Using a spatula, loosen the outside and inside edges of the pan and remove cake.

Variation

Turn this into a daffodil cake by folding in 2 tbsp (25 mL) grated lemon zest and 1 tbsp (15 mL) grated orange zest with the dry ingredients. Drizzle wedges of cake with lots of lemon sauce.

Caramel Apple Cake

SERVES 12 TO 15

Just one small piece of this moist delight will have you craving more! No need for frosting — the topping bakes right on.

Tips

Wrap individual pieces and freeze, then grab a piece when you're packing your lunch. It will be perfectly thawed by noon.

We used Fuji apples, but you can choose any baking variety; there's no need to peel.

Half of an 8-oz (225 g) package of toffee bits yields ³/₄ cup (175 mL). They are found in the baking aisle with chocolate chips and dried fruit at major grocery stores.

13- by 9-inch (3 L) baking pan, lightly greased and bottom lined with parchment paper

1¼ cups	sorghum flour	300 mL
½ cup	quinoa flour	125 mL
⅓ cup	tapioca starch	75 mL
2 tsp	xanthan gum	10 mL
1½ tsp	GF baking powder	7 mL
1 tsp	baking soda	5 mL
¼ tsp	salt	1 mL
1 tsp	ground cinnamon	5 mL
½ cup	butter, softened	125 mL
¾ cup	packed brown sugar	175 mL
2	eggs	2
1 cup	plain yogurt	250 mL
1 tsp	vanilla	5 mL
2 cups	diced apples	500 mL
¾ cup	toffee bits	175 mL

TOPPING

⅓ cup	sorghum flour	75 mL
2 tbsp	packed brown sugar	25 mL
¼ cup	cold butter, cubed	50 mL
¾ cup	toffee bits	175 mL
½ cup	white chocolate chips	125 mL

1. In a large bowl or plastic bag, combine the sorghum flour, quinoa flour, tapioca starch, xanthan gum, baking powder, baking soda, salt and cinnamon. Mix well and set aside.

2. In another large bowl, using an electric mixer, cream the butter and brown sugar until well combined. Add eggs and beat until light and fluffy. Beat in yogurt and vanilla until blended. Gradually mix in dry ingredients, mixing just until smooth, about 2 minutes. Stir in apples and toffee bits. Spoon into prepared pan. Using a moistened rubber spatula, spread to edges and smooth top. Let stand for 30 minutes. Meanwhile, preheat oven to 350°F (180°C).

3. *Prepare the topping:* In a small bowl, stir together sorghum flour and brown sugar. Using a pastry blender or two knives, cut in butter until mixture resembles coarse crumbs. Stir in toffee bits and white chocolate chips. Sprinkle topping over the batter. Do not pack.

4. Bake in preheated oven for 30 to 35 minutes, or until a cake tester inserted in the center comes out clean. Let cool in the pan on a rack for 10 minutes. Remove from pan, quickly remove parchment and let cool completely, topping side up, on a rack.

Variation

Substitute an equal amount of chopped pecans for the toffee bits in both the cake and topping, and an equal amount of ground ginger for the cinnamon in the cake only. Your family will never recognize this as the same recipe.

Orange Hazelnut Bundt Cake

Not too big, not too sweet, but just right to finish off a weekday meal — and perfect to take along to your next casual neighborhood get-together.

Tips

To chop the hazelnuts, pulse in a food processor only until the nuts are coarsely chopped. Don't worry: the nuts will not be uniform in size.

Set a kitchen timer for 3 minutes when beating. You will be surprised by how long 3 minutes seems.

It is worth the effort to zest the fresh orange and then juice it for the best orange flavor. First, zest the orange cold from the refrigerator, then warm orange in the microwave on High for 30 seconds and roll it on the counter to loosen the juice.

Substitute almond or pecan flour for the hazelnut flour and almonds or pecans for the chopped hazelnuts.

10-inch (3 L) Bundt pan, lightly greased

¾ cup	amaranth flour	175 mL
⅔ cup	hazelnut flour	150 mL
⅔ cup	sorghum flour	150 mL
⅓ cup	potato starch	75 mL
1½ tsp	xanthan gum	7 mL
2 tsp	GF baking powder	10 mL
¾ tsp	baking soda	4 mL
½ tsp	salt	2 mL
½ cup	butter or shortening, softened	125 mL
¾ cup	granulated sugar	175 mL
3	eggs	3
2 tbsp	grated orange zest	25 mL
⅔ cup	freshly squeezed orange juice	150 mL
1 tsp	almond extract	5 mL
1 cup	coarsely chopped hazelnuts	250 mL
	Simple Hot Fudge Sauce (see recipe, page 157)	

1. In a large bowl or plastic bag, combine the amaranth flour, hazelnut flour, sorghum flour, potato starch, xanthan gum, baking powder, baking soda and salt. Mix well and set aside.

2. In another large bowl, using an electric mixer, cream butter and sugar until well combined. Add eggs, one at a time, and cream until light and fluffy. Stir in orange zest and juice and almond extract. Add dry ingredients and beat on medium for 3 minutes. Fold in hazelnuts. Spoon into prepared pan. Using a moistened rubber spatula, spread to edges and smooth top. Let stand for 30 minutes. Meanwhile, preheat oven to 350°F (180°C).

3. Bake in preheated oven for 40 to 50 minutes, or until a cake tester inserted in the center comes out clean. Let cake cool in the pan on a rack for 10 minutes. Remove from pan and let cool completely on a rack. Drizzle with Simple Hot Fudge Sauce.

Peach Cheesecake

Baskets of peaches ready at the market, family reunion coming soon — put these together for a memorable dessert.

Tips

Use enough fruit to cover the base generously and finish a whole piece of fruit.

When peaches are not in season, use about 2 cups (500 mL) well-drained canned peach slices.

Ultra low-fat cream cheese or fat-free cream cheese should not be substituted for regular in baked cheesecakes. However, light cream cheese can be used.

When using a dark-colored springform pan, decrease the oven temperature by 25°F (20°C).

Cheesecake can be made up to 1 month in advance. Cool completely, then wrap whole cheesecake or individual slices tightly and freeze until ready to serve. Thaw in refrigerator and garnish just before serving.

Preheat oven to 325°F (160°C)
8-inch (20 cm) springform pan

BASE AND TOPPING

2¼ cups	Gingerbread Crumbs (see recipe, page 154)	550 mL
2 tbsp	melted butter	25 mL
3 to 4	peaches, peeled and thickly sliced	3 to 4

CHEESECAKE

2	packages (each 8 oz/250 g) light or regular cream cheese, softened	2
¼ cup	packed brown sugar	50 mL
1 tbsp	grated lemon zest	15 mL
2 tbsp	freshly squeezed lemon juice	25 mL
3	eggs	3
1 cup	GF sour cream	250 mL

1. Center springform pan on a large square of foil and press foil up the sides of the pan.
2. *Prepare the base:* In a bowl, combine Gingerbread Crumbs and butter; mix well. Set aside ½ cup (125 mL) to use for the topping. Press remainder of crumbs into bottom of prepared pan. Refrigerate until chilled, about 15 minutes. Arrange the peaches over the chilled base.
3. *Prepare the cheesecake:* In a large bowl, using an electric mixer, beat cream cheese until smooth. Slowly add brown sugar, lemon zest and juice. Beat until light and fluffy. Add eggs one at a time, beating well after each. Stir in sour cream. Pour over the peach-lined base.
4. *Add the topping:* Sprinkle reserved crumb mixture over filling.
5. Bake in preheated oven for 65 to 70 minutes, or until center is just set. Let cool to room temperature in pan on a rack. Cover and refrigerate overnight before serving.

Pecan Roulade

SERVES 8 TO 10

This rich rolled sponge cake, filled with a knockout Mocha Buttercream, is sure to become the centerpiece of your next dessert buffet. It's great to have one in the freezer for last-minute entertaining.

Tips

For better volume when beating egg whites, make sure the bowl and beaters are completely free of grease. Wash right before using them.

Wrapped airtight, the roulade can be frozen for up to 1 month.

For instructions on toasting nuts, see Techniques Glossary, page 181.

For instructions on warming egg whites to room temperature, see Techniques Glossary, page 179.

Wrap airtight and freeze for up to 1 month. Thaw, wrapped, in refrigerator.

Preheat oven to 375°F (190°C)
13- by 9-inch (3 L) baking pan, bottom lined with parchment paper

2 cups	Mocha Buttercream (see recipe, page 151), chilled for at least 3 hours	500 mL
2 tbsp	pecan flour	25 mL
2 tbsp	cornstarch	25 mL
1/3 cup	unsweetened cocoa powder, sifted	75 mL
1 cup	coarsely chopped pecans, toasted	250 mL
4	egg whites, at room temperature (see tip, at left)	4
1/4 tsp	cream of tartar	1 mL
1/4 cup	granulated sugar	50 mL
4	egg yolks	4
Pinch	salt	Pinch
2 tbsp	brandy	25 mL
	GF confectioner's (icing) sugar	

1. Prepare Mocha Buttercream at least 3 hours ahead to allow time to chill.
2. In a small bowl or plastic bag, combine pecan flour, cornstarch, cocoa and pecans. Set aside.
3. In a large bowl, using an electric mixer with wire whisk attachment, beat egg whites until foamy. While beating, add cream of tartar. Continue to beat until egg whites are stiff. Gradually add sugar and continue beating until mixture is very stiff and glossy but not dry. Set aside.
4. In a small bowl, using an electric mixer, beat egg yolks and salt until thick and lemon-colored, approximately 5 minutes. Stir in brandy.
5. Fold egg yolk mixture into egg whites. Sprinkle half the cocoa mixture over the whites and fold in gently. Repeat with remaining half. Spoon into prepared pan and carefully spread evenly to the edges.

Substitute an equal amount of thawed, frozen orange juice concentrate for the brandy in both the roulade and the buttercream.

6. Bake in preheated oven for 7 to 10 minutes, or until top springs back when lightly touched. Let cool in the pan on a rack for 10 minutes.

7. Dust lightly with confectioner's sugar. Loosen edges of cake with a knife. Turn out onto a clean, lint-free towel set on a cooling rack; carefully remove parchment paper. Starting at the long side, immediately roll up cake in the tea towel. Let cool completely on a rack.

8. Gently unroll cake, being careful not to flatten it, and spread with Mocha Buttercream. Roll up again and place seam side down on a serving platter. Cover and refrigerate for 30 to 60 minutes, until chilled, or for up to 1 day.

Mocha Buttercream

Chocolate and coffee — partners in crime! This is the perfect filling for Pecan Roulade or frosting for any layer cake.

Tip
To avoid lumps, sift confectioner's (icing) sugar and cocoa together.

2 cups	GF confectioner's (icing) sugar	500 mL
1/3 cup	unsweetened cocoa powder	75 mL
2 tsp	instant coffee granules	10 mL
1/2 cup	butter, softened	125 mL
3 tbsp	brandy	45 mL

1. In a bowl, sift together confectioner's sugar, cocoa and coffee granules; add butter and brandy. Using an electric mixer, beat for approximately 5 minutes, or until light and fluffy.

Variation
To make chocolate buttercream, omit the instant coffee granules.

Trendy Pastry

1½ cups	sorghum flour	375 mL
1 cup	cornstarch	250 mL
½ cup	tapioca starch	125 mL
1 tbsp	granulated sugar	15 mL
2 tsp	GF baking powder	10 mL
1 tsp	salt	5 mL
1	egg	1
½ cup	ice water	125 mL
⅓ cup	vegetable oil	75 mL
2 tbsp	cider vinegar	25 mL

People today are concerned about what type of fat they're eating. This recipe is in answer to a request for pastry made with vegetable oil. Though not quite as tender as that made with shortening or butter, this pastry is just as easy to work with.

Tips

If the pastry cracks while you're handling it, don't worry: just use the excess to patch.

This pastry can also be made into tart shells to fill with custard and fresh fruit or to make mini-quiches or hors d'oeuvre tartlets.

You can freeze the pastry for up to 3 months. Thaw in refrigerator. Bring to room temperature before rolling out.

While rolling out the first half of the dough, cover remaining half to prevent it from drying out.

Food Processor Method

1. In a food processor fitted with a metal blade, pulse sorghum flour, cornstarch, tapioca starch, sugar, baking powder and salt until mixed. Set aside.
2. In a small bowl, whisk together egg, ice water, oil and vinegar.
3. With food processor running, add egg mixture through feed tube in a slow, steady stream. Process until dough just holds together. Do not let it form a ball.

Traditional Method

1. In a large bowl, sift sorghum flour, cornstarch, tapioca starch, sugar, baking powder and salt. Set aside.
2. In a small bowl, whisk together egg, ice water, oil and vinegar.
3. Stirring with a fork, sprinkle egg mixture, a little at a time, over the flour mixture to make a soft dough.

For Both Methods

4. Divide dough in half. Gently gather each piece into a ball and flatten into a disc. Place the pastry disc between two sheets of parchment paper. Using quick, firm strokes of the rolling pin, roll out the dough into a circle about 1-inch (2.5 cm) larger than the diameter of the inverted pie plate. Carefully remove the top sheet of parchment paper and invert the pastry over the pie plate, easing it in. Carefully peel off the remaining sheet of parchment paper.

5. To prepare another single-crust pie, repeat Step 4 with the remaining dough. To prepare the top crust for a double-crust pie, roll out the remaining dough as directed above, then set aside.

For a Single-Crust Pie

Trim excess pastry to edge of pie plate, patch any cracks with trimmings, and press edges with a fork. Or, for a more attractive finish, using a sharp knife, trim the pastry evenly, leaving a 1-inch (2.5 cm) overhang. Tuck pastry under to form a raised double rim. Flute or crimp the edges.

To Bake an Unfilled Pastry Shell

To prevent pastry from shrinking or puffing up, prick bottom and sides with a fork. Bake in oven preheated to 425°F (220°C) for 18 to 20 minutes, or until golden. Let cool completely before filling.

To Bake a Filled Pastry Shell

Do not prick the pastry. Spoon filling into unbaked pastry shell and bake according to individual recipe directions.

For a Double-Crust Pie

For instructions on finishing and baking, see recipe for Strawberry Rhubarb Pie, page 155.

Gingerbread Crumbs

**MAKES ABOUT
8 CUPS (2 L)**

*Our crumb crust, made
from these crumbs, is
the perfect flavor partner
for Peach Cheesecake
(see recipe, page 149)
and Praline Pumpkin
Delight (see recipe,
page 168).*

Tips

Store crumbs in an
airtight freezer bag at
room temperature for up
to 2 weeks or freeze for
up to 3 months.

Spreading batter to an
even thickness ensures
the center is cooked
before the edges become
too dark.

Bake the two pans at the
same time, in the top
and bottom thirds of the
oven; switch and rotate
the pans halfway through
the baking time.

Recipe can be doubled
to make 16 cups (4 L)
so you'll always have
crumbs at the ready.

Substitute garbanzo-fava
(garfava) bean flour or
whole bean flour for the
chickpea flour.

Preheat oven to 325°F (160°C)
Two 15- by 10-inch (40 by 25 cm) jelly-roll pans, lightly greased

1²/₃ cups	sorghum flour	400 mL
1 cup	chickpea (garbanzo bean) flour	250 mL
1/3 cup	tapioca starch	75 mL
1 tsp	xanthan gum	5 mL
1 tsp	baking soda	5 mL
1/2 tsp	salt	2 mL
2 tsp	ground ginger	10 mL
1 tsp	ground cinnamon	5 mL
1/2 tsp	ground cloves	2 mL
1 cup	shortening or butter, softened	250 mL
3/4 cup	granulated sugar	175 mL
1 cup	fancy molasses	250 mL
2	eggs	2

1. In a large bowl or plastic bag, combine sorghum flour, chickpea flour, tapioca starch, xanthan gum, baking soda, salt, ginger, cinnamon and cloves; set aside.

2. In another large bowl, using an electric mixer, cream shortening, sugar, molasses and eggs. Slowly beat in dry ingredients until combined. Using a moistened rubber or metal spatula, spread half the dough in each prepared pan. Remoisten spatula when the batter begins to stick to it.

3. Bake in preheated oven for 20 minutes. Let cool completely in pans on a rack. Break into pieces, then pulse a few pieces at a time in a food processor until crumb consistency.

Strawberry Rhubarb Pie

We can hardly wait until fresh local rhubarb and strawberries are both at their prime, to enjoy our yearly feast of crisps, cobblers and pies.

Tips

For the best flavor and color, purchase fresh local berries while they're in season. Choose firm stalks of rhubarb that are fresh and crisp; slender stalks are more tender than thick ones.

No time to roll out a top crust? Form the entire recipe of dough into one large disc. On a rimless baking sheet, roll out dough into a 17-inch (43 cm) circle, leaving edge uneven. Leaving a 4-inch (10 cm) border, spoon filling into the center. Fold pastry border over the filling, leaving fruit exposed in the center. Bake in oven preheated to 425°F (220°C) for 10 minutes. Reduce heat to 375°F (190°C) and bake for 50 to 60 minutes more, or until crust is golden and filling is bubbly. Let cool on sheet on a rack.

9-inch (23 cm) deep-dish pie plate

4 cups	chopped (1-inch/2.5 cm) fresh rhubarb (or frozen rhubarb, thawed)	1 L
2 cups	quartered fresh strawberries	500 mL
1 cup	granulated sugar	250 mL
1/3 cup	tapioca starch	75 mL
2 tsp	freshly squeezed lemon juice	10 mL
	Trendy Pastry (see recipe, page 152)	

1. In a large bowl, toss together rhubarb, strawberries, sugar and tapioca starch. Add the lemon juice. Let stand for 15 minutes. Meanwhile, preheat oven to 425°F (220°C).

2. Roll out pastry for a double-crust pie and press the bottom pastry into pie plate as directed on pages 152–53. Spoon filling into the unbaked pie shell and moisten the edge. Carefully remove the top sheet of parchment paper from the top pastry, invert and cover the filling. Carefully peel off the remaining sheet of parchment paper. Trim pastry, leaving a 3/4-inch (2 cm) overhang. Fold overhang under bottom pastry rim, seal and flute edge.

3. Make numerous 1/2-inch (1 cm) slits near the center of the pie through the crust to the filling or cut out a 1-inch (2.5 cm) circle in the center of the crust.

4. Position the oven racks to divide the oven into thirds. Place a baking sheet on the bottom rack to catch the drips if pie boils over. Bake in preheated oven on the top rack for 20 minutes. Reduce heat to 350°F (180°C) and bake for 40 to 50 minutes, or until crust is golden and filling is bubbly. Shield edges with foil if they are browning too quickly. Let cool completely on a rack.

Variation

To make a rhubarb pie, substitute rhubarb for the strawberries and increase the granulated sugar to 1 1/4 cups (300 mL).

Pear Almond Torte

This is a thin torte that does not rise much. No fancy pastry-making techniques required here: it is prepared completely in the food processor. Serve warm from the oven or cold straight from the fridge.

Tips

To quickly peel pears, use a vegetable peeler.

Torte can be made up to 2 days ahead. Cover with plastic wrap and refrigerate.

A ripe pear will yield slightly when you apply gentle thumb pressure near the base of the stem. Ripen pears in a paper bag on the counter. Check daily — ripening may take 1 to 6 days.

If desired, drizzle torte with Simple Hot Fudge Sauce (see recipe, page 157).

9-inch (23 cm) springform pan, lightly greased and dusted with rice flour

TOPPING

2 tsp	granulated sugar	10 mL
1 tsp	ground cinnamon	5 mL
1/2 tsp	ground nutmeg	2 mL
2	pears, peeled, cored and cut into eighths	2
1/3 cup	slivered almonds	75 mL

BASE

1/2 cup	almond flour	125 mL
1/2 cup	brown rice flour	125 mL
1 tsp	xanthan gum	5 mL
2 tsp	GF baking powder	10 mL
1/4 tsp	salt	1 mL
1/2 cup	butter, softened	125 mL
1 cup	granulated sugar	250 mL
1 tsp	almond extract	5 mL
2	eggs	2

1. *Prepare the topping:* In a medium bowl, stir together sugar, cinnamon and nutmeg; add pears and toss until evenly coated; set aside.

2. *Prepare the base:* In a small bowl, combine almond flour, rice flour, xanthan gum, baking powder and salt until mixed; set aside.

3. In the bowl of a food processor fitted with the metal blade, pulse the butter, sugar and almond extract until smooth and creamy; scrape down sides. Add eggs, one at a time, pulsing just until mixed. Add flour mixture; pulse until mixed. Scrape batter into prepared pan. Spread to edges and smooth top with a moist rubber spatula.

4. Arrange the coated pear wedges in a circle over the batter and sprinkle with almonds. Let stand for 30 minutes. Meanwhile, preheat oven to 325°F (160°C).

5. Bake in preheated oven for 50 to 55 minutes, or until top is a rich golden color and a cake tester inserted in the center comes out clean. Transfer to a rack. Run a knife around the inside edge of pan. Let stand 10 minutes, then remove ring. Serve warm or let cool completely on base on rack.

> **Variation**
>
> In season, substitute apples, plums, peaches or apricots for the pears. Use enough fruit to cover the base generously and finish a whole piece of fruit.

Simple Hot Fudge Sauce

MAKES ½ CUP (125 ML)

Drizzle this quick sauce over Pear Almond Torte, ice cream, fresh fruit or anything that chocolate improves.

Tips

Timing in the microwave is critical. If you heat the sauce for too long, it could seize.

Stir like crazy. It'll take about 2 to 3 minutes.

Substitute flavored chocolate chips for regular chocolate chips.

½ cup	chocolate chips	125 mL
2 to 3 tbsp	milk	25 to 45 mL

1. In a small microwave-safe bowl, microwave chocolate chips and milk, uncovered, on High for 30 seconds, or until partially melted. Stir until completely melted.

> **Variation**
>
> For a richer sauce, substitute half-and-half (10%) cream, whipping (35%) cream or evaporated milk for the milk.

Chocolate Lover's Hazelnut Surprise

These individual decadent chocolate delights are a close relative of the molten lava cake, oozing with bittersweet chocolate and hazelnut liqueur. Serve garnished with fresh strawberries or raspberries in season.

Tips

One individually wrapped square of baking chocolate weighs 1 oz (30 g).

For instructions on warming eggs to room temperature, see Techniques Glossary, page 179.

Baking time is critical; even one extra minute will cause the center to become solid instead of molten and the top crust to burn.

We tried to make this dessert with 1/2-cup (125 mL) dishes without success. Your ramekins are the correct size if they hold 3/4 cup (175 mL) water when full to the top.

Preheat oven to 450°F (220°C)
Six 3/4-cup (175 mL) ramekins or ceramic soufflé dishes

2 tsp	butter, softened	10 mL
2 tsp	unsweetened cocoa powder	10 mL
8 oz	bittersweet chocolate, chopped	250 g
1/2 cup	butter	125 mL
2 tbsp	hazelnut flour	25 mL
2 tbsp	sorghum flour	25 mL
1/2 tsp	xanthan gum	2 mL
4	eggs, at room temperature	4
1/2 cup	GF confectioner's (icing) sugar	125 mL
2 tbsp	hazelnut liqueur	25 mL

1. Using a scrunched-up piece of waxed paper, lightly butter the bottom and sides of ramekins. Coat bottom and sides with cocoa.

2. In a large microwave-safe bowl, microwave chocolate and butter, uncovered, on Medium (50%) for 3 minutes, or until partially melted. Stir until completely melted. Let cool to room temperature.

3. In a small bowl, combine hazelnut flour, sorghum flour and xanthan gum. Set aside.

4. In a large bowl, using an electric mixer, beat eggs, confectioner's sugar and liqueur until thick and lemon-colored, approximately 8 minutes. (Set a kitchen timer, as 8 minutes seems like forever.) With mixer on low, add cooled melted chocolate; continue beating until combined. Add dry ingredients and beat just until blended. Ladle into each ramekin and place on baking sheet.

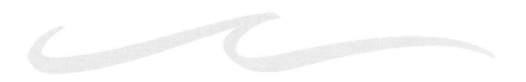

Garnish with large white chocolate curls. To make curls, peel room-temperature chocolate firmly along its length with a sharp vegetable peeler.

For easier cleanup, allow ramekins to soak in hot soapy water.

Substitute an equal amount of coffee liqueur or cold double-strength coffee for the hazelnut liqueur.

You can also serve the "Surprise" right in the ramekins, topped with chopped toasted hazelnuts (see Techniques Glossary, page 181, for instructions on toasting nuts). Ramekins should still be hot from the oven when you serve.

5. Bake immediately or refrigerate for up to 4 hours. Remove from refrigerator to bring to room temperature (approximately 45 minutes) before baking. Bake in preheated oven for 11 minutes, or until "Surprise" is puffed and crusted, but center is still soft. Let cool on a rack for 3 minutes. Run a knife around the inside edge of each ramekin to loosen. Cover with individual dessert plates and invert. Remove hot ramekin. Serve immediately. (Ramekins can be left on for up to 20 minutes before removing for serving.)

Blueberry Almond Dessert

Anne Lindsay, PHEc, a cookbook author known for her healthy-eating recipes, told us this is her most popular recipe. With Anne's permission, we have developed a gluten-free version for you. This soft, creamy dessert is delicious with its hint of almond flavor in the crust and topping.

Tips

This dessert can be made ahead, covered with plastic wrap and refrigerated for up to 2 days.

When using frozen blueberries, there is no need to defrost.

Substitute fresh or frozen cranberries, or a berry mix, for the blueberries.

Add $1/8$ to $1/4$ tsp (0.5 to 1 mL) ground mace for a slightly different flavor.

To make one large flan, double the recipe and bake base in a 9-inch (23 cm) springform pan for 15 to 18 minutes. Add topping and bake for a further 60 to 65 minutes.

Preheat oven to 325°F (160°C)
Six $3/4$-cup (175 mL) ramekins or ceramic soufflé dishes, lightly buttered

BASE

$1/3$ cup	almond flour	75 mL
$1/3$ cup	amaranth flour	75 mL
$1/4$ cup	granulated sugar	50 mL
1 tsp	GF baking powder	5 mL
$1/2$ tsp	xanthan gum	2 mL
Pinch	salt	Pinch
1	egg white	1
3 tbsp	cold butter, cut into 1-inch (2.5 cm) cubes	45 mL
$1/2$ tsp	almond extract	2 mL
2 cups	fresh or frozen blueberries	500 mL

TOPPING

$1/3$ cup	granulated sugar	75 mL
2 tbsp	tapioca starch	25 mL
1	egg, lightly beaten	1
1 cup	plain yogurt	250 mL
$1 1/2$ tsp	grated lemon zest	7 mL
$1/4$ tsp	almond extract	1 mL
$3/4$ cup	sliced almonds	175 mL

1. *Prepare the base:* In a food processor fitted with a metal blade, pulse the almond flour, amaranth flour, sugar, baking powder, xanthan gum and salt. Add egg white, butter and almond extract; pulse until dough forms a ball. Divide among prepared ramekins. Do not press down.

2. Bake in preheated oven for 10 to 12 minutes, just until light golden. Sprinkle blueberries over hot base.

3. *Prepare the topping:* In a small bowl, using an electric mixer, combine sugar and tapioca starch. Add egg, yogurt, lemon zest and almond extract and mix until smooth. Pour over blueberries. Sprinkle with almonds.

4. Bake in preheated oven for 20 minutes, or until top is set. Let cool to room temperature in ramekins on a rack before serving or refrigerating.

Almond Sponge Cake (page 145)

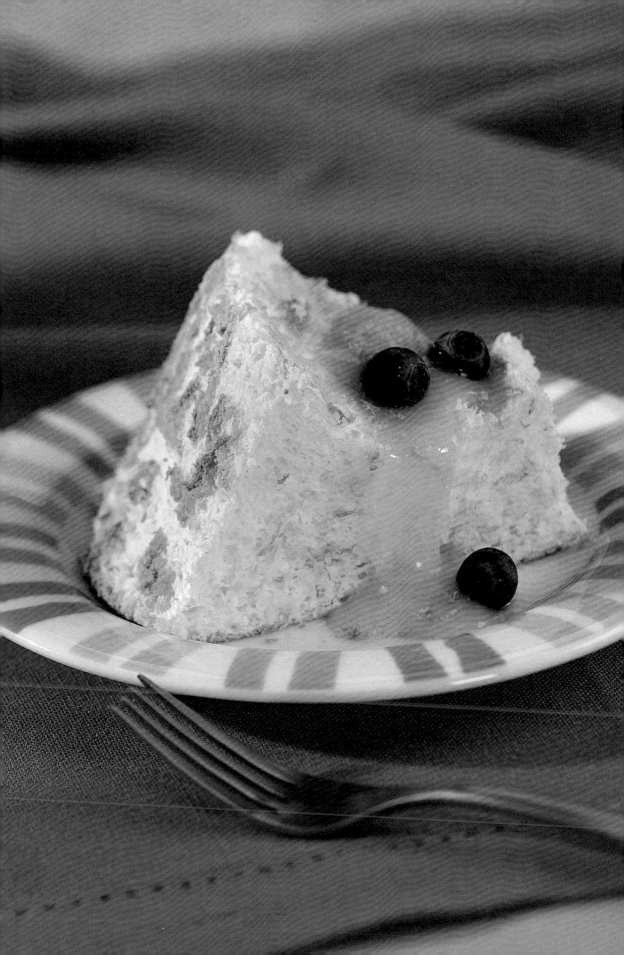

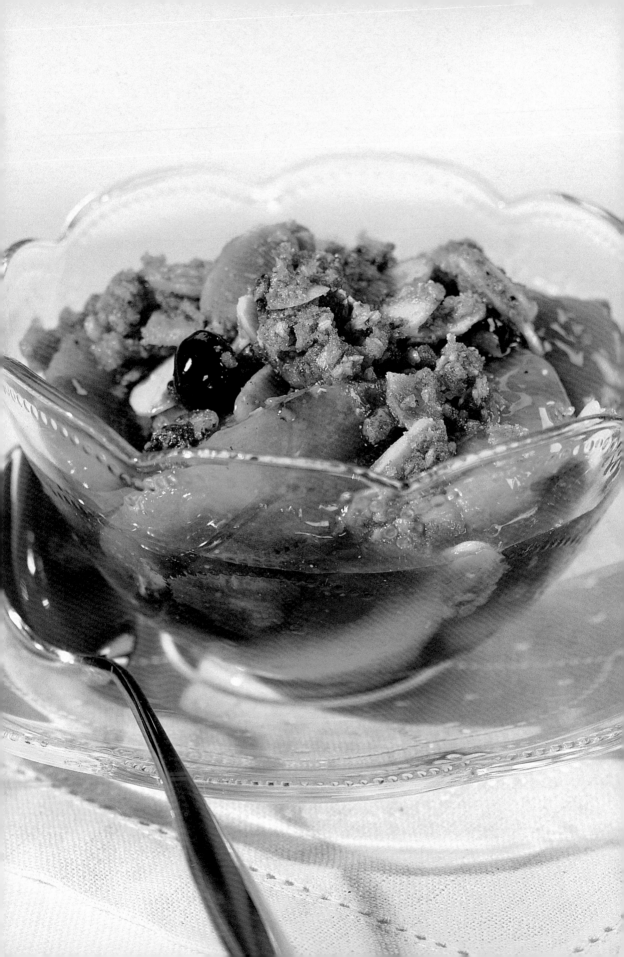

Blueberry Peach Crisp

SERVES 6 TO 8

Late summer means peaches are plentiful and evenings are cool — time to make this comfort food.

Tips

5 large or 7 small peaches yield 4 cups (1 L) sliced.

To increase the fiber, leave the peel on the peaches.

For a crisper topping, cover with foil for the first half of the baking time.

Check with the manufacturer to be sure buckwheat flakes are gluten-free.

If using frozen fruit, there is no need to defrost before using; just increase the baking time until fruit is fork-tender.

Instead of baking, microwave, uncovered, on High for 4 minutes. Turn dish one-quarter turn and microwave on High for 3 to 4 minutes longer, or until fruit is tender. Let stand for 5 minutes.

Substitute nectarines for the peaches.

Recipe can be divided in half and baked in a lightly greased 9- by 5-inch (2 L) loaf pan.

Blueberry Peach Crisp (this page)

Preheat oven to 375°F (190°C)
8-cup (2 L) casserole dish, lightly greased

TOPPING

⅓ cup	sorghum flour	75 mL
⅓ cup	whole bean flour	75 mL
¼ cup	packed brown sugar	50 mL
1 tbsp	grated orange zest	15 mL
½ tsp	ground nutmeg	2 mL
⅓ cup	melted butter	75 mL
¾ cup	GF buckwheat flakes	175 mL
½ cup	sliced almonds	125 mL

BASE

4 cups	sliced fresh peaches	1 L
1 cup	fresh or frozen blueberries	250 mL
¼ cup	cornstarch	50 mL
2 tbsp	granulated sugar	25 mL

1. *Prepare the topping:* In a medium bowl, combine sorghum flour, whole bean flour, brown sugar, orange zest and nutmeg. Drizzle with melted butter and mix until crumbly. Add buckwheat flakes and almonds. Set aside.
2. *Prepare the base:* In prepared casserole dish, combine peaches, blueberries, cornstarch and sugar.
3. Sprinkle topping over the fruit. Do not pack.
4. Bake in preheated oven for 20 to 25 minutes, or until fruit is bubbly and topping is browned. Serve warm.

Chocolate-Glazed Pavlova

Pavlova is an Australian dessert named for the Russian ballerina, Anna Pavlova. It consists of a crisp crunchy meringue exterior and a creamy marshmallow interior shell filled with whipped cream and mounded with fresh fruit. Try our alternative lighter filling.

Tips

This is an ideal time to use liquid egg whites, available in cartons. Use $1/2$ cup (125 mL) for this recipe.

If berry (castor or fruit/instant dissolving) sugar is not available, use granulated sugar. Add very slowly.

Make sure the mixer bowl and beaters are completely free of grease. Plastic tends to retain grease more readily than metal or glass.

For instructions on warming egg whites to room temperature, see Techniques Glossary, page 179.

For instructions on whipping cream and toasting nuts, see Techniques Glossary, page 181.

Preheat oven to 275°F (140°C)
Baking sheet, lined with parchment paper

MERINGUE

4	egg whites, at room temperature (see tips, at left)	4
$1/4$ tsp	cream of tartar	1 mL
1 cup	berry (castor or fruit/instant dissolving) sugar	250 mL
1 tbsp	cornstarch	15 mL
1 tsp	white vinegar	5 mL

FILLING

1 cup	whipping (35%) cream	250 mL
2 cups	sliced mixed fruit, such as peaches, kiwi and strawberries	500 mL

ALTERNATIVE FILLING

4 oz	light cream cheese, softened	125 g
$1/3$ cup	GF confectioner's (icing) sugar	75 mL
Dash	almond extract	Dash
2 cups	sliced mixed fruit, such as peaches, kiwi and strawberries	500 mL

GLAZE

1 oz	semi-sweet chocolate, chopped	30 g
$1/2$ tsp	vegetable oil	2 mL
$3/4$ cup	toasted slivered almonds	175 mL

1. Using a pencil, draw an 8-inch (20 cm) circle in the center of the parchment (you can trace an 8-inch/20 cm cake pan or cardboard circle). Flip parchment over.

2. *Prepare the meringue:* In a large glass or metal bowl, using an electric mixer, beat egg whites and cream of tartar until soft peaks form. Gradually beat in berry sugar, a little at a time, until stiff, glossy peaks form. Fold in cornstarch and vinegar. Spoon the meringue to fill the circle on the parchment paper. Using the back of a large metal spoon, lightly smooth top.

3. Bake in preheated oven for 60 to 75 minutes, or until crisp and lightly browned but still soft in the middle. Turn off oven; let stand in oven 1 hour to dry. Remove from oven and invert onto a large serving plate. Meringue will deflate in the center. Let cool completely.

4. *Prepare the filling:* In a small bowl, using an electric mixer, whip cream until soft peaks form. Spread over meringue shell to within 1 inch (2.5 cm) of the edge. Top with fresh fruit.

5. *Prepare the glaze:* In a small microwave-safe bowl, microwave chocolate and oil, uncovered, on Medium (50%) for 1 to 2 minutes, or until chocolate is partially melted. Stir until completely melted. Drizzle in ribbons over fruit and sprinkle with toasted almonds.

Alternative Filling

1. In a small bowl, using an electric mixer, beat cream cheese, confectioner's sugar and almond extract until light and fluffy. Spread over meringue shell to within 1 inch (2.5 cm) of the edge. Top with fresh fruit.

Variation

Make eight 4-inch (10 cm) individual meringues. Spoon mixture into mounds and spread each into a 4-inch (10 cm) circle or heart shape, heaping mixture at edges to form a nest. Bake for 45 minutes. Let stand in oven, with oven turned off, for 45 minutes.

Hot Apple Crêpes

This make-ahead dessert can be assembled at the last minute for your next dinner party.

Tips

For more information about making crêpes and storing crêpes made in advance, see page 25.

1¹/₂ lbs (750 g) of apples yield 6 cups (1.5 L) sliced.

You can also prepare the apple filling in the microwave: In a large microwave-safe bowl, microwave butter, uncovered, on High for 1 minute, or until melted. Add apples, brown sugar and cinnamon and microwave, uncovered, on High, for 2 to 4 minutes, stirring once or twice, or until apples are just tender.

Apple filling can be stored in the refrigerator in an airtight container for up to 4 days. To reheat, microwave on Medium (50%) for 2 to 4 minutes.

6-inch (15 cm) crêpe pan or nonstick skillet, lightly greased

CRÊPES

¹/₄ cup	amaranth flour	50 mL
¹/₄ cup	chickpea (garbanzo bean) flour	50 mL
2 tbsp	potato starch	25 mL
2 tsp	granulated sugar	10 mL
¹/₂ tsp	xanthan gum	2 mL
¹/₂ tsp	salt	2 mL
2	eggs	2
²/₃ cup	milk	150 mL
¹/₃ cup	water	75 mL
1 tbsp	melted butter	15 mL

APPLE FILLING

¹/₃ cup	butter	75 mL
³/₄ cup	packed brown sugar	175 mL
6 cups	thickly sliced apples	1.5 L
1¹/₂ tsp	ground cinnamon	7 mL

GF vanilla-flavored yogurt

1. *Prepare the crêpes:* In a large bowl or plastic bag, mix together amaranth flour, chickpea flour, potato starch, sugar, xanthan gum and salt.
2. In a small bowl, whisk together eggs, milk, water and melted butter. Pour mixture over dry ingredients all at once, whisking until smooth. Cover and refrigerate for at least 1 hour or for up to 2 days. Bring batter back to room temperature before making crêpes.

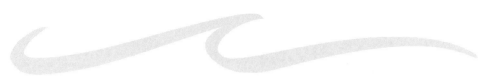

Substitute 2 cups
(500 mL) of your
favorite prepared GF
fruit pie filling for the
apple filling.

Substitute whipped
cream, GF frozen yogurt
or GF ice cream for the
GF yogurt.

3. Heat prepared pan over medium heat; add 3 to 4 tbsp
   (45 mL to 50 mL) batter for each crêpe, tilting and
   rotating pan to ensure batter covers entire bottom.
   Cook for 1 to 1½ minutes, or until edges begin to
   brown. Turn carefully with a non-metal spatula. Cook
   for another 30 to 45 seconds, or until bottom is dotted
   with brown spots. Remove to a plate and repeat with
   remaining batter.

4. *Prepare the apple filling:* In a saucepan, melt butter over
   medium heat. Add brown sugar, apples and cinnamon
   and simmer gently for 4 to 6 minutes, or until apples
   are just tender.

5. *Assemble the crêpes:* Spoon an equal portion of hot
   apple filling down the center of each crêpe. Roll and
   serve seam side down, topped with GF vanilla yogurt.

Crêpes Suzette

Soaked in orange and brandy, then flambéed at the table, these crêpes are sure to impress your guests. Only you need to know that they are gluten-free.

Tips

Brandy flames easily when warmed to body temperature before lighting.

For more information about making crêpes and storing crêpes made in advance, see page 25.

Any orange liqueur can be used in this recipe — Grand Marnier, Cointreau or Triple Sec.

6-inch (15 cm) crêpe pan or nonstick skillet, lightly greased

CRÊPES

¼ cup	amaranth flour	50 mL
¼ cup	chickpea (garbanzo bean) flour	50 mL
2 tbsp	potato starch	25 mL
2 tsp	granulated sugar	10 mL
½ tsp	xanthan gum	2 mL
½ tsp	salt	2 mL
2	eggs	2
⅔ cup	milk	150 mL
⅓ cup	water	75 mL
1 tbsp	melted butter	15 mL
1 tbsp	grated orange zest	15 mL

ORANGE SAUCE

½ cup	butter	125 mL
½ cup	frozen orange juice concentrate, thawed	125 mL
½ cup	orange-flavored liqueur	125 mL
4 tsp	granulated sugar	20 mL
¼ cup	brandy	50 mL

1. *Prepare the crêpes:* In a large bowl or plastic bag, mix together amaranth flour, chickpea flour, potato starch, sugar, xanthan gum and salt.

2. In a small bowl, whisk together eggs, milk, water, melted butter and orange zest. Pour mixture over dry ingredients all at once, whisking until smooth. Cover and refrigerate for at least 1 hour or for up to 2 days. Bring batter back to room temperature before making crêpes.

3. Heat prepared pan over medium heat; add 3 to 4 tbsp (45 mL to 50 mL) batter for each crêpe, tilting and rotating pan to ensure batter covers entire bottom. Cook for 1 to $1\frac{1}{2}$ minutes, or until edges begin to brown. Turn carefully with a non-metal spatula. Cook for another 30 to 45 seconds, or until bottom is dotted with brown spots. Remove to a plate and repeat with remaining batter.

4. *Prepare the orange sauce:* In a nonstick skillet or crêpe pan, melt butter over medium heat. Add orange juice, orange liqueur and sugar.

5. Add a crêpe and spoon sauce over crêpe until well saturated. Gently fold crêpe in half and then into quarters. Gently remove to a heatproof dish and keep warm. Repeat with remaining crêpes. Pour any remaining sauce over crêpes.

6. In a small saucepan, over medium-low heat, warm the brandy just until heated through but not boiling. Remove from heat. Using a long match, ignite brandy; immediately pour over crêpes in dish. Serve 2 to 3 crêpes per person.

Praline Pumpkin Delight

*Crave pumpkin pie?
With a moist texture,
subtle spiciness and the
crunch of pecans, this is
an excellent dessert to
serve everyone.*

Tips

Just like any custard, this
one is done when a knife
blade inserted in the
center comes out clean.

If pan appears to be
getting too full or too
heavy to lift, pour in only
two-thirds of the filling.
Then, after pan is set on
oven rack, pour in the
remaining filling to within
$1/2$ inch (1 cm) of the top.

If using a dark nonstick
springform pan, lower the
oven temperature to 350°F
(180°C) and decrease the
baking time to 50 to
60 minutes.

This dessert can be
made ahead, covered
and refrigerated for
up to 2 days.

Don't add more caramel
sauce than is called for;
if you do, the base will
become brittle and
impossible to cut, and
you may not be able
to remove the side
of the pan.

Preheat oven to 375°F (190°C)
9-inch (23 cm) springform pan

PRALINE BASE

1¼ cups	Gingerbread Crumbs (see recipe, page 154)	425 mL
2 tbsp	melted butter	25 mL
1 cup	pecan halves or pieces	250 mL
½ cup	GF caramel sauce (see tip, at left)	125 mL

PUMPKIN FILLING

4	eggs	4
1	can (14 oz/385 mL) 2% evaporated milk	1
2 cups	pumpkin purée (not pie filling)	500 mL
⅔ cup	packed brown sugar	150 mL
2 tsp	ground cinnamon	10 mL
1 tsp	ground allspice	5 mL
1 tsp	ground ginger	5 mL
1 tsp	salt	5 mL

1. *Prepare the praline base:* In a small bowl, combine Gingerbread Crumbs and butter; mix well. Press crumbs into bottom of pan. Sprinkle with pecans. Bake in preheated oven for 6 to 8 minutes, or until pecans are toasted. Immediately drizzle with caramel sauce, leaving a 1-inch (2.5 cm) circle around the edge. Let cool to room temperature.

2. *Prepare the pumpkin filling:* In a large bowl, using an electric mixer, combine eggs, evaporated milk, pumpkin purée, brown sugar, cinnamon, allspice, ginger and salt.

3. Holding a large spoon or spatula over the praline base, slowly pour the pumpkin filling over the spoon and let drizzle into pan (this prevents the filling from disturbing the base). (If there is too much filling for the springform pan, pour the excess into a lightly greased ovenproof casserole dish and bake for 15 to 20 minutes, until set.)

4. Bake in preheated oven for 60 to 70 minutes, or until filling is set. Let cool to room temperature in pan on a rack before serving.

Sticky Date Pudding

We all know how the British love their puddings, often called "puds." Donna fell in love with this one on a recent holiday in the British Isles. The traditional way to serve it is warm with a warm toffee sauce. We've adapted it for you to enjoy. So will we!

Tips

When purchasing chopped dates, check for wheat starch in the coating.

Instead of chopping dates with a knife, simply snip with scissors. When scissors become sticky, dip in hot water.

Pudding can be wrapped airtight and frozen for up to 2 months, and individual pieces can be defrosted in the microwave on Medium (50%) for 2 to 4 minutes, or until warm.

Serve with warm Nutmeg Rum Sauce (see recipe, page 170) instead of Toffee Sauce.

Preheat oven to 350°F (180°C)
9-inch (2.5 L) square baking pan, lightly greased

½ cup	sorghum flour	125 mL
½ cup	whole bean flour	125 mL
¼ cup	tapioca starch	50 mL
1½ tsp	GF baking powder	7 mL
1 tsp	xanthan gum	5 mL
Pinch	salt	Pinch
1 cup	coarsely chopped pitted dates	250 mL
1 cup	water	250 mL
1 tsp	baking soda	5 mL
¼ cup	butter, softened	50 mL
¾ cup	packed brown sugar	175 mL
1 tsp	vanilla	5 mL
2	eggs	2
	Toffee Sauce (see recipe, page 170)	

1. In a large bowl or plastic bag, mix together sorghum flour, whole bean flour, tapioca starch, baking powder, xanthan gum and salt; set aside.

2. In a small saucepan, combine dates and water and bring to a boil over high heat. Reduce heat to medium-low and simmer until softened, about 5 minutes. Remove from heat and add baking soda; stir until foaming stops. Let cool to room temperature.

3. In a large bowl, using an electric mixer, cream butter. Gradually add brown sugar and beat for 2 minutes, until light and fluffy. Using a rubber spatula, scrape the bottom and sides of the bowl. Beat in vanilla; add eggs one at a time, beating for 2 minutes after each. Stir in date mixture and dry ingredients. Combine well. Spoon batter into prepared pan. Using a moistened rubber spatula, spread to edges and smooth top.

4. Bake in preheated oven for 25 to 35 minutes, or until cake tester inserted in the center comes out clean. Let pudding cool in the pan on a rack for 10 minutes. Remove from pan and serve warm with warm Toffee Sauce.

Nutmeg Rum Sauce

MAKES 1¼ CUPS (300 mL)

Serve this delightful sauce over Almond Sponge Cake (see recipe, page 145) or Sticky Date Pudding (see recipe, page 169).

Tip
Substitute brandy or cold coffee for the rum.

1 cup	packed brown sugar	250 mL
½ cup	2% evaporated milk	125 mL
1 tsp	ground nutmeg	5 mL
½ cup	butter	125 mL
2 tbsp	dark rum	25 mL

1. In a saucepan, combine brown sugar, evaporated milk and nutmeg. Bring to a rolling boil over medium heat, stirring constantly. Reduce heat to low and simmer for 2 to 3 minutes. Remove from heat and add butter and rum, stirring until butter melts. Serve hot.

Toffee Sauce

MAKES 1¼ CUPS (300 mL)

This buttery sweet sauce is best when served warm. Try drizzling it over ice cream.

Tip
We like to not just drizzle but drench warm Sticky Date Pudding (see recipe, page 169) with this sauce.

½ cup	packed brown sugar	125 mL
½ cup	butter	125 mL
¼ cup	liquid honey	50 mL
¼ cup	2% evaporated milk	50 mL

1. In a small saucepan, combine brown sugar, butter and honey. Heat gently over low heat, stirring constantly, until the sugar dissolves. Simmer for 2 to 3 minutes, or until sauce thickens and bubbles. Stir in evaporated milk and remove from heat.

Storing and Reheating Sauces

Sauces can be refrigerated for up to 1 week. Reheat in a saucepan over medium-low heat, stirring occasionally, or microwave, uncovered, on High for a few seconds.

Sauces can be frozen for up to 2 months. They stay soft enough to scoop out in small quantities. Warm in the microwave on Medium (50%) for 1 to 2 minutes.

Appendix: Thickener Substitutions

Starches	To thicken 1 cup (250 mL) of liquid	Cooking precautions	Cooked appearance	Tips
Arrowroot	2 tbsp (25 mL)	• add during last 5 minutes of cooking • stir only occasionally • do not boil	• clear shine • glossier than cornstarch	• thickens at a lower temperature than cornstarch • not as firm as cornstarch when cool • doesn't break down as quickly as cornstarch • more expensive • separates when frozen
Cornstarch	2 tbsp (25 mL)	• stir constantly • boil gently for only 1 to 3 minutes	• translucent and shiny	• thickens as it cools • boiling too rapidly causes thinning • boiling for more than 7 minutes causes thinning • add acid (lemon juice) after removing from heat
Potato starch	1 tbsp (15 mL)	• stir constantly	• more translucent and clearer than cornstarch	• lumps easily • thickest at boiling point • thickens as it cools • separates when frozen
Tapioca starch (cassava)	3 tbsp (45 mL)	• add during last 5 minutes of cooking • stir constantly	• transparent and shiny	• dissolves more easily than cornstarch • firms more as it cools • best to use for freezing
Flours	**To thicken 1 cup (250 mL) of liquid**	**Cooking precautions**	**Cooked appearance**	**Tips**
Amaranth flour	3 tbsp (45 mL)	• browns quickly and could burn if not watched carefully • thickens at boiling point and slightly more after 5 to 7 minutes of boiling • reheats in microwave	• golden brown color • cloudy, opaque • smooth	• nutty, beefy aroma • if too thick, can be thinned with extra liquid • reheats • excellent for gravy
Bean flour	3 tbsp (45 mL)	• thickens after 2 to 3 minutes of boiling • does not thicken with extra cooking	• warm tan color • cloudy, opaque • smooth	• can be used for sauces • brown in hot fat to a golden color
Rice flour (brown or white)	2 tbsp (25 mL)	• dissolve in cold liquid rather than hot fat or pan drippings • thickens after 5 to 7 minutes of boiling • continues to thicken with extra cooking	• opaque, cloudy • grainy texture • bland flavor	• thickens more as it cools • thickens rapidly when reheated and stirred • stable when frozen
Sorghum flour	2 tbsp (25 mL)	• thickens after 2 to 3 minutes of boiling • does not thicken with extra cooking	• dull • similar to wheat flour	• doesn't thin or thicken with excess cooking • thickens as it cools • reheats well on stove-top or microwave • thickens quickly when extra is added
Sweet rice flour	2 tbsp (25 mL)	• thickens after 5 to 8 minutes of boiling	• shiny, opaque • grainy texture • bland flavor	• thickens as it cools

Equipment Glossary

Bundt pan. A tube pan with fluted sides.

Cake tester. A thin, long wooden or metal stick or wire attached to a handle that is used for baked products to test for doneness.

Cooling rack. Parallel and perpendicular thin bars of metal at right angles, with feet attached, used to hold hot baking off the surface to allow cooling air to circulate.

Crêpe pan. Smooth, low, round pan with a heavy bottom and sloping sides. It ranges from 5 to 7 inches (13 to 18 cm) in diameter.

Dutch oven. A large deep pot with a tight-fitting lid, used for stewing or braising.

Griddle. Flat metal surface on which food is cooked. Can be built into a stove or stand-alone.

Grill. Heavy rack set over a heat source used to cook food, usually on a propane, natural gas or charcoal barbecue.

Jelly-roll pan. A rectangular baking pan, 15 by 10 by 1 inch (40 by 25 by 2.5 cm), used for baking thin cakes.

Loaf pan. Metal container used for baking loaves. Common pan sizes are 9 by 5 inches (2 L) and 8 by 4 inches (1.5 L). Danish loaf pans measure 12 by 4 by $2\frac{1}{2}$ inches (30 by 10 by 6 cm).

Mandolin(e). A manually operated slicer with adjustable blades. The food is held at a 45-degree angle and is passed and pressed against the blade to produce uniform pieces of different thickness, either straight-cut or rippled.

Parchment paper. Heat-resistant paper similar to waxed paper, usually coated with silicon on one side; used with or as an alternative to other methods (such as applying vegetable oil or spray) to prevent baked goods from sticking to the baking pan. Sometimes labeled "baking paper."

Pastry blender. Used to cut solid fat into flour, it consists of five metal blades or wires held together by a handle.

Pastry brush. Small brush with nylon or natural bristles used to apply glazes or egg washes to dough. Wash thoroughly after each use. To store, lay flat or hang on a hook through a hole in the handle.

Pizza wheel. A large, sharp-edged wheel (without serrations) anchored to a handle.

Ramekins. Usually sold as a set of small, deep, straight-sided ceramic soufflé dishes also known mini-bakers. Used to bake individual servings of a pudding, cobbler or custard. Capacity ranges from 4 oz or $\frac{1}{2}$ cup (125 mL) to 8 oz. or 1 cup (250 mL).

Rolling pin. A heavy, smooth cylinder of wood, marble, plastic or metal; used to roll out dough.

Skewer. A long, thin stick (made of wood or metal) used in baking to test for doneness.

Spatula. A utensil with a handle and blade that can be long or short, narrow or wide, flexible or inflexible. It is used to spread, lift, turn, mix or smooth foods. Spatulas are made of metal, rubber or plastic.

Springform pan. A circular baking pan, available in a range of sizes, with a separable bottom and side. The side is removed by releasing a clamp, making the contents easy to remove.

Thermometers.

- *Instant-read thermometer.* Bakers use this metal-stemmed instrument to test the internal temperature of baked products such as cakes and breads. Stem must be inserted at least 2 inches (5 cm) into the food for an accurate reading. When yeast bread is baked, it should register 200°F (100°C).

- *Meat thermometer.* Used to read internal temperature of meat. Temperatures range from 120°F to 200°F (60°C to 100°C). Before placing meat in the oven, insert the thermometer into the thickest part, avoiding the bone and gristle. (If using an instant-read thermometer, remove meat from oven and test with thermometer. For more information, see Digital instant-read thermometer in Techniques Glossary, page 179.)

- *Oven thermometer.* Used to measure temperatures from 200°F to 500°F (100°C to 260°C). It either stands on or hangs from an oven rack.

Tube pan. A deep round pan with a hollow tube in the center, usually 10 inches (25 cm) in diameter, 16 cups (4 L) volume.

Zester. A tool used to cut very thin strips of outer peel from citrus fruits. It has a short, flat blade tipped with five small holes with sharp edges. Another style of zester that is popular is made of stainless steel and looks like a tool found in a workshop used for planing wood.

Ingredient Glossary

Almond. Crack open the shell of an almond, and you will find an ivory-colored nut encased in a thin brown skin. With the skin removed (see Techniques Glossary, page 178), the almond is called blanched. In this form, almonds are sold whole, sliced, slivered and ground. Two cups (500 mL) almonds weigh about 12 oz (375 g).

Almond flour (almond meal). See Nut flour in The Gluten-Free Bakeshop Revisited, page 9. For instructions on how to make, see Nut flour in Techniques Glossary, page 181.

Almond paste. Made of ground blanched almonds, sugar and egg whites, almond paste is coarser, darker and less sweet then marzipan. Do not substitute one for the other.

Amaranth flour. See The Gluten-Free Bakeshop Revisited, page 8.

Arborio rice. Oval Italian short-grain rice with a distinct nutty flavor and a hard core. It has the ability to absorb large quantities of liquid, and becomes creamy when cooked. Traditionally, it is used for risotto, and we like it for rice pudding.

Arrowroot. Referred to as a starch, as a flour and as arrowroot starch flour. (See also The Gluten-Free Bake Shop Revisited, page 8.)

Asiago cheese. A pungent grayish-white hard cheese from northern Italy. Cured for more than 6 months, its texture is ideal for grating.

Baking chips. Similar in consistency to chocolate chips, but with different flavors such as butterscotch, peanut butter, cinnamon and lemon. Check to make sure they are gluten-free.

Baking powder. Select gluten-free baking powder. A chemical leavener, containing an alkali (baking soda) and an acid (cream of tartar), that gives off carbon dioxide gas under certain conditions.

Baking soda (sodium bicarbonate). A chemical leavener that gives off carbon dioxide gas in the presence of moisture — particularly acids such as lemon juice, buttermilk and sour cream. It is also one of the components of baking powder.

Bean flour. See The Gluten-Free Bake Shop Revisited, page 8.

Bell peppers. The sweet-flavored members of the capsicum family (which include chilies and other hot peppers), these peppers have a hollow interior lined with white ribs and seeds attached at the stem end. They are most commonly green, red or yellow, but can also be white or purple.

Bird's eye chili peppers. Small, very hot chilis that are highly pungent. Use them to add "pure heat" to a meal without very much of the chili favor coming through. The heat level is 9 on a scale of 1 to 10.

Black bean flour. A high-fiber gluten-free flour used mainly in Tex-Mex dishes.

Blueberries. Wild low-bush berries are smaller than the cultivated variety and more time-consuming to pick, but their flavor makes every minute of picking time worthwhile. Readily available year-round in the frozen fruit section of many grocery stores.

Brown rice flour. See Rice flour in The Gluten-Free Bake Shop Revisited, page 9.

Brown sugar. A refined sugar with a coating of molasses. It can be purchased coarse or fine and comes in three varieties: dark, golden and light.

Buckwheat. Also known as saracen corn. Not related, despite its name, to wheat (which is a grain), buckwheat is the seed of a plant from the rhubarb family. Buckwheat flour is dark with a strong pungent flavor and is gluten-free. Buckwheat groats are the hulled seeds of the buckwheat plant. These seeds are soft and white with a mild flavor; when roasted or toasted, the flavor intensifies. Roasted whole buckwheat, called kasha, has a strong nutty flavor and chewy texture. It is low in fat and cholesterol-free.

Buckwheat flakes (oatmeal style). These small brittle flakes have the appearance of small rolled oats with a slightly sweeter flavor and a slightly browner color; they can replace oatmeal in crisps, meatloaves and squares.

Butter. A spread produced from dairy fat and milk solids, butter is interchangeable with shortening, oil or margarine in most recipes.

Buttermilk. Named for the way in which it was originally produced — that is, from milk left in the churn after the solid butter was removed — buttermilk is now made with fresh, pasteurized milk that has been cultured (or soured) with the addition of a bacterial culture. The result is a slightly thickened dairy beverage with a salty, sour flavor similar to yogurt. Despite its name, buttermilk is low in fat.

Caraway seeds. These small, crescent-shaped seeds of the caraway plant have a nutty, peppery, licorice-like flavor.

Cardamom. This popular spice is a member of the ginger family. A long green or brown pod contains the strong, spicy, lemon-flavored seed. Although native to India, cardamom is used in Middle Eastern, Indian and Scandinavian cooking — in the latter case, particularly for seasonal baked goods.

Cassava. See Tapioca starch in The Gluten-Free Bake Shop Revisited, page 10.

Castor or caster sugar. A finely granulated sugar, used in beverages and frostings, that dissolves rapidly due to its smaller crystal size. It is also known as berry or superfine sugar. Regular granulated sugar may be substituted on a one-to-one basis.

Cheddar cheese. Always select an aged, or old, good-quality Cheddar for baking recipes. (The flavor of mild or medium Cheddar is not strong enough for baking.) Weight/volume equivalents are:

4 oz (125 g) = 1 cup (250 mL) grated;
2 oz (60 g) = 1/2 cup (125 mL) grated;
1 1/2 oz (45 g) = 1/3 cup (75 mL) grated.

Coconut. The fruit of a tropical palm tree, with a hard woody shell that is lined with a hard white flesh. There are three dried forms available, which can be sweetened or not: flaked, shredded and the smallest, desiccated (thoroughly dried).

Corn flour. A flour that can be milled from the entire kernel of corn. Corn flour and cornstarch are not interchangeable in recipes. Freeze corn flour to prevent molds from developing.

Cornmeal. The dried ground kernels of white, yellow or blue corn. It has a gritty texture and is available in coarse, medium and fine grind. It is the coarser grind of corn flour and cornstarch. Check labels of commercial products for addition of wheat. Maizemeal can be corn or wheat. Its starchy-sweet flavor is most commonly associated with cornbread — a regional specialty of the southern United States.

Cornstarch. See The Gluten-Free Bake Shop Revisited, page 8.

Corn syrup. A thick, sweet syrup made from cornstarch, sold in clear (light) or brown (dark or golden) varieties. The latter has caramel flavor and color added.

Cranberry. Grown in bogs on low vines, these sweet-tart berries are available fresh, frozen and dried. Fresh cranberries are available only in season — typically from mid-October until January, depending on your location — but can be frozen right in the bag. Substitute dried cranberries for sour cherries, raisins or currants.

Cream of tartar. Used to give volume and stability to beaten egg whites, cream of tartar is also an acidic component of baking powder. Tartaric acid is a fine white crystalline powder that forms naturally during the fermentation of grape juice on the inside of wine barrels.

Cross-contamination. The process by which one product comes in contact with another one that is to be avoided. For example, toasters, oven mitts, cutting boards and knives, when used for products containing gluten, still have gluten on them, which is passed on to the gluten-free product. You must either have separate tools or be sure that the gluten is washed off completely before being used by people with gluten sensitivity.

Currants. Similar in appearance to small dark raisins, currants are made by drying a special seedless variety of grape. Not the same as a type of berry that goes by the same name.

Dates. The fruit of the date palm tree, dates are long and oval in shape, with a paper-thin skin that turns from green to dark brown when ripe. Eaten fresh or dried, dates have a very sweet, light brown flesh around a long, narrow seed.

Eggs. Liquid egg products, such as Naturegg Simply Whites®, Break Free® and Omega Pro® liquid eggs and Just Whites®, are available in Canada and the United States. Powdered egg whites such as Just Whites® can be used by reconstituting with warm water or as a powder. A similar product is called meringue powder in Canada. Substitute 2 tbsp (25 mL) liquid egg product for each white of a large egg.

Egg replacer. A powder used in place of eggs that acts as a leavening agent. Reconstitute according to package instructions.

Egg substitute. A liquid made from egg whites, or dried egg whites reconstituted according to package instructions.

Evaporated milk. A milk product with 60% of the water removed. It is sterilized and canned, which gives it a cooked taste and darker color.

Fava bean flour. See Bean flour in The Gluten-Free Bake Shop Revisited, page 8.

Feta cheese. A crumbly white Greek-style cheese with a salty, tangy flavor. Store in the refrigerator, in its brine, and drain well before using. Traditionally made with sheep's or goat's milk in Greece and usually with cow's milk in Canada and the U.S.

Fig. A pear-shaped fruit with a thick, soft skin, available in green and purple. Eaten fresh or dried, the tan-colored sweet flesh contains many tiny edible seeds.

Filbert. See Hazelnut.

Flaxseed. Thin and oval, dark brown in color, flaxseed adds a crunchy texture to baked products. Research indicates that flaxseed can aid in lowering blood cholesterol levels. Ground flaxseed (also known as linseed) stales quickly. It acts as a tenderizer for yeast breads. It can be used with or without eggs and adds omega-3 fatty acids and fiber. Flaxseed should be cracked or ground to be digested. Whole flaxseed can be stored at room temperature for up to 1 year. Ground flaxseed can be stored in the refrigerator for up to 90 days, although for optimum freshness it is best to grind it as you need it.

Garbanzo bean flour. See Bean flour in The Gluten-Free Bake Shop Revisited, page 8.

Garbanzo-fava flour. See Bean flour in The Gluten-Free Bake Shop Revisited, page 8.

Garfava flour. See Bean flour in The Gluten-Free Bake Shop Revisited, page 8.

Garlic. An edible bulb composed of several sections (cloves), each covered with a papery skin. An essential ingredient in many styles of cooking.

Ginger. A bumpy rhizome, ivory to greenish-yellow in color, with a tan skin. Fresh gingerroot has a peppery, slightly sweet flavor, similar to lemon and rosemary, and a pungent aroma. Ground ginger is made from dried gingerroot. It is spicier and not as sweet or as fresh. Crystallized or candied ginger is made from pieces of fresh gingerroot that have been cooked in sugar syrup and coated with sugar.

Gluten. A natural protein in wheat flour that becomes elastic with the addition of moisture and kneading. Gluten traps gases produced by leaveners inside the dough and causes it to rise.

Glutinous rice flour. See Rice flour in The Gluten-Free Bake Shop Revisited, page 9.

Golden raisins. See Raisins.

Granulated sugar. A refined, crystalline white form of sugar that is also commonly referred to as "table sugar" or just "sugar."

Guar gum. A white flour-like substance made from an East Indian seed high in fiber, this vegetable substance contains no gluten. It may have a laxative effect for some people. It can be substituted for xanthan gum.

Half-and-half cream. The lightest of all creams, it is half milk, half cream and has a butterfat content between 10% and 18%. It can't be whipped, but is used with coffee or on cereal. To substitute, use equal parts cream and milk *or* evaporated milk *or* $^7/_8$ cup (210 mL) milk plus $1^1/_2$ tbsp (22 mL) butter or margarine.

Hazelnut. Also known as filberts, hazelnuts have a rich, sweet flavor that complements ingredients such as coffee and chocolate. Remove the bitter brown skin before using.

Hazelnut flour (Hazelnut meal). See Nut flour in The Gluten-Free Bakeshop Revisited, page 9. For instructions on how to make, see Nut flour in Techniques Glossary, page 181.

Hazelnut liqueur. The best known is Frangelico, a hazelnut-flavored liqueur made in Italy.

Hemp hearts®. Shelled hemp seeds. Due to their high fat content, hemp hearts should be purchased in small amounts and stored in the refrigerator (can be stored for up to 90 days). Can be eaten raw or added to baking.

Herbs. See also individual herbs. Plants whose stems, leaves or flowers are used as a flavoring, either dried or fresh. To substitute fresh herbs for dried, a good rule of thumb is to use three times the amount of fresh as dried. Taste and adjust the amount to suit your preference.

Honey. Sweeter than sugar, honey is available in liquid, honeycomb and creamed varieties. Use liquid honey for baking.

Kalamata olives. See Olives (Kalamata).

Kasha. See Buckwheat.

Linseed. See Flaxseed.

Maple syrup. A very sweet, slightly thick brown liquid made by boiling the sap from North American maple trees. Use pure maple syrup, not pancake syrup, in baking.

Marzipan. A sweet nut paste made from ground almonds, sugar and egg whites. Used as candy filling and for cake decorations, it is sweeter and lighter in color than almond paste. Do not substitute one for the other.

Margarine. A solid fat derived from one or more types of vegetable oil. Do not use lower-fat margarines in baking, as they contain too much added water.

Mesclun. A mixture of small, young, tender salad greens such as spinach, frisée, arugula, oak leaf and radicchio. Also known as salad mix, spring mix or baby greens and sold prepackaged or in bulk in the grocery produce section.

Millet. The small seed of a cereal grass or grain closely related to corn. With a nutty aroma and taste, it is an excellent source of fiber and a moderate source of protein.

Molasses. A byproduct of refining sugar, molasses is a sweet, thick, dark brown (almost black) liquid. It has a distinctive, slightly bitter flavor and is available in fancy and blackstrap varieties. Use the fancy variety for baking unless blackstrap is specified. Store in the refrigerator if used infrequently.

Nonfat dry milk. See Skim milk powder.

Nut flour (nut meal). See The Gluten-Free Bakeshop Revisited, page 9.

Olives (Kalamata). A large, flavorful variety of Greek olive, typically dark purple in color and pointed at one end. They are usually sold packed in olive oil or vinegar.

Olive oil. Produced from pressing tree-ripened olives. Extra-virgin oil is taken from the first cold pressing; it is the finest and fruitiest, pale straw to pale green in color, with the least amount of acid, usually less than 1%. Virgin oil is taken from a subsequent pressing; it contains 2% acid and is pale yellow. Light oil comes from the last pressing; it has a mild flavor, light color and up to 3% acid. It also has a higher smoke point. Product sold as "pure olive oil" has been cleaned and filtered; it is very mild-flavored and has up to 3% acid.

Parsley. A biennial herb with dark green curly or flat leaves used fresh as a flavoring or garnish. It is also used dried in soups and other mixes. Substitute parsley for half the amount of a strong-flavored herb such as basil.

Pea flour. See The Gluten-Free Bake Shop Revisited, page 9.

Pecan. The nut of the hickory tree, pecans have a reddish-mahogany shell and beige flesh. They have a high fat content and are a milder-flavored alternative to walnuts.

Pecan flour (pecan meal). See Nut flour in The Gluten-Free Bakeshop Revisited, page 9. For instructions on how to make, see Nut flour in Techniques Glossary, page 181.

Pistachio nut. Inside a hard, tan-colored shell, this pale green nut has a waxy texture and a mild flavor.

Poppy seeds. The tiny round blue-gray seed of the poppy has a sweet, nutty flavor. Often used as a garnish or as a topping for a variety of breads.

Potato flour. See Potato starch in The Gluten-Free Bake Shop Revisited, page 9.

Potato starch (potato starch flour). See The Gluten-Free Bake Shop Revisited, page 9.

Pumpkin seeds. Hulled and roasted green pumpkin seeds have a nutty flavor that enhances many breads. In Mexico, where they are eaten as a snack and used as a thickener in cooking, they are also known as pepitas.

Quinoa flour. See The Gluten-Free Bakeshop Revisited, page 9.

Rhubarb. A perennial plant with long, thin red- to pink-colored stalks resembling celery and large green leaves. Only the tart-flavored stalks are used for cooking, as the leaves are poisonous. For 2 cups (500 mL) cooked rhubarb, you will need 3 cups (750 mL) chopped fresh, about 1 lb (500 g).

Raisins. Dark raisins are sun-dried Thompson seedless grapes. Golden raisins are treated with sulphur dioxide and dried artificially, yielding a moister, plumper product. Muscat, a grape grown throughout the Mediterranean region, Australia and California, is used for eating and making raisins and wine. Both Muscat and Lexia are large, flat seeded raisins.

Rice bran. See The Gluten-Free Bake Shop Revisited, page 9.

Rice flour. See The Gluten-Free Bake Shop Revisited, page 9.

Rice polish. See The Gluten-Free Bake Shop Revisited, page 9.

Sambal oelek (Thai chili paste). An Indonesian flavoring paste made from ground bird's eye chilis, salt, oil and vinegar. Popular in Indonesian/Asian cuisines.

Sesame seeds. Small, flat, oval seeds that have a rich, nut-like flavor when roasted. Purchase the tan (hulled), not black (unhulled), variety for use in baking.

Shortening. A partially hydrogenated, solid, white flavorless fat made from vegetable sources.

Skim milk powder. The dehydrated form of fluid skim milk. Use 1/4 cup (50 mL) skim milk powder for every 1 cup (250 mL) water.

Sorghum flour. See The Gluten-Free Bake Shop Revisited, page 9.

Sour cream. A thick, smooth, tangy product made by adding bacterial cultures to pasteurized, homogenized cream containing varying amounts of butterfat. Check the label: some lower-fat and fat-free brands may contain gluten.

Soy flour. See The Gluten-Free Bake Shop Revisited, page 10.

Starch. Starch is found in the cells of plants and is insoluble in cold water. When cooked, the granules swell and thicken or gel.

Sugar substitute. For baking, the best choice is sucralose, which is made from processed sugar and remains stable at any temperature.

Sun-dried tomatoes. Available either dry or packed in oil, sun-dried tomatoes have a dark red color, a soft chewy texture and a strong tomato flavor. Use dry, not oil-packed, sun-dried tomatoes in recipes. Use scissors to snip.

Sunflower seeds. Use shelled, unsalted, unroasted sunflower seeds in bread recipes. If only roasted salted seeds are available, rinse under hot water and dry well before using.

Sweet peppers. See Bell peppers.

Sweet potato. A tuber with orange flesh that stays moist when cooked. Not the same as a yam, although yams can substitute for sweet potatoes in recipes.

Sweet rice flour. See Rice flour in The Gluten-Free Bake Shop Revisited, page 9.

Tapioca starch (tapioca flour). See The Gluten-Free Bake Shop Revisited, page 10.

Tarragon. An herb with narrow, pointed, dark green leaves and a distinctive anise-like flavor with undertones of sage. Use fresh or dried.

Vegetable oil. Common oils used are corn, sunflower, safflower, olive, canola, peanut and soy.

Walnuts. A sweet-fleshed nut with a large wrinkled shell.

Wild rice. In its natural state, wild rice is gluten-free, but when found in boxed wild rice/white rice mixes, it's best avoided. For instructions on how to cook, see Techniques Glossary, page 181.

Xanthan gum. A natural carbohydrate made from a microscopic organism called *Xanthomonas campestris*, this gum is produced from the fermentation of glucose. It is used to add volume and viscosity to baked goods. As an ingredient in gluten-free baking, it gives the dough strength, allowing it to rise and preventing it from being too dense in texture. It does not mix with water, so must be combined with dry ingredients. Purchase from bulk or health food stores.

Yeast. A tiny single-celled organism that, given moisture, food and warmth, creates gas that is trapped in bread dough, causing it to rise. Bread machine yeast (instant yeast) is added directly to the dry ingredients of bread. We use this yeast rather than active dry as it does not need to be activated in water before using. Store in the freezer in an airtight container for up to 2 years.

Yogurt. Made by fermenting cow's milk using a bacteria culture. Plain yogurt is gluten-free, but not all flavored yogurt is.

Zest. Strips from the outer layer of rind (colored part only) of citrus fruit. Avoid the bitter part underneath. Used for its intense flavor.

Techniques Glossary

Almonds. *To blanch:* Cover almonds with boiling water and let stand, covered, for 3 to 5 minutes. Drain. Grasp the almond at one end, pressing between your thumb and index finger, and the nut will pop out of the skin. Nuts are more easily chopped or slivered while still warm from blanching. *To toast:* see Nuts.

Almond flour (almond meal). *To make:* See Nut flour.

Baking pan. *To prepare or to grease:* Either spray the bottom and sides of the baking pan with nonstick cooking spray or brush with a pastry brush or a crumpled-up piece of waxed paper dipped in vegetable oil or shortening.

Bananas. *To mash and freeze:* Select overripe fruit, mash and package in 1 cup (250 mL) amounts in freezer containers. Freeze for up to 6 months. Defrost and warm to room temperature before using. About 2 to 3 medium bananas yield 1 cup (250 mL) mashed.

Barbecue by indirect method. To cook with the heat source coming from one or both sides of the food and not from directly beneath it.

Beat. To stir vigorously to incorporate air using a spoon, whisk, handheld beater or electric mixer.

Black beans. *To cook:* For every 1 cup (250 mL) dried black beans, cover with 3 cups (750 mL) cold water. Bring to a boil for 2 minutes; cover and let stand for 1 hour. Drain. Add 6 cups (1.5 L) cold water and boil uncovered until tender, approximately 1 hour.

Blanch. To completely immerse food in boiling water and then quickly in cold water, to loosen and easily remove skin, for example.

Blend. To mix two or more ingredients together thoroughly, with a spoon or using the low speed of an electric mixer.

Bread crumbs. *To make fresh:* For best results, the GF bread should be at least 1 day old. Using the pulsing operation of a food processor or blender, process until crumbs are of the desired consistency. *To make dry:* Spread bread crumbs in a single layer on a baking sheet and bake at 350°F (180°C) for 6 to 8 minutes, shaking pan frequently, until lightly browned, crisp and dry. (Or microwave, uncovered, on High for 1 to 2 minutes, stirring every 30 seconds.) *To store:* Package in airtight containers and freeze for up to 3 months.

Cake crumbs. See Bread crumbs.

Cast-iron skillet. *To clean:* Add 2 tbsp (25 mL) salt to a dry cast-iron skillet. Rub with an old toothbrush. Keep replacing salt until it remains white. This usually requires 2 to 3 applications of salt and about 5 minutes.

Chocolate. *To melt:* Chop each 1 oz (30 g) square into 4 to 6 pieces. Place in a heat-proof bowl or the top of a double-boiler over hot water to partially melt the chocolate. Remove from heat and continue stirring until completely melted.

Coconut. *To toast:* See Nuts.

Combine. To stir two or more ingredients together for a consistent mixture.

Cream. To combine softened fat and sugar by beating to a soft, smooth creamy consistency while trying to incorporate as much air as possible.

Cream cheese. *To warm quickly to room temperature:* For each 8-oz (250 g) package, cut into 1-inch (2.5 cm) cubes, arrange in a circle on a microwave-safe plate and microwave on High for 1 minute.

Cut in. To combine solid fat and flour until the fat is the size required (for example, the size of small peas or meal). Use either two knives or a pastry blender.

Digital instant-read thermometer. *To test meat for doneness:* Insert the metal stem of the thermometer at least 2 inches (5 cm) into the thickest part of cooked chicken, fish, pork, beef, etc. For thin cuts, it may be necessary to insert the thermometer horizontally. Meatballs can be stacked. *To test baked goods for doneness:* Insert the metal stem of the thermometer at least 2 inches (5 cm) into the thickest part of baked good. Temperature should register 200°F (100°C).

Dredge. To coat a food with flour or bread crumbs before frying, enabling batter to adhere to the food more easily.

Drizzle. To slowly spoon or pour a liquid (such as frosting or melted butter) in a very fine stream over the surface of food.

Dust. To coat by sprinkling GF confectioner's (icing) sugar, cocoa powder or any GF flour lightly over food or a utensil.

Eggs. *To warm to room temperature:* Place eggs in the shell from the refrigerator in a bowl of hot water and let stand for 5 minutes.

Egg whites. *To warm to room temperature:* Separate eggs while cold. Place bowl of egg whites in a larger bowl of hot water and let stand for 5 minutes. *To whip to soft peaks:* Beat to a thickness that comes up as the beaters are lifted and folds over at the tips. *To whip to stiff peaks:* Beat past soft peaks until the peaks remain upright when the beaters are lifted.

Egg yolks. *To warm to room temperature:* Separate eggs while cold. Place bowl of egg yolks in a larger bowl of hot water and let stand for 5 minutes.

Flaxseed. *To grind:* Place whole seeds in a coffee grinder or blender. Grind only the amount required. If necessary, store extra ground flaxseed in the refrigerator. *To crack:* Pulse in a coffee grinder, blender or food processor just long enough to break the seed coat but not long enough to grind completely.

Fold. To gently combine light, whipped ingredients with heavier ingredients without losing the incorporated air. Using a rubber spatula, gently fold in a circular motion. Move down one side of the bowl and across the bottom, fold up and over to the opposite side and down again, turning bowl slightly after each fold.

Garlic. *To roast:* Cut off top of head to expose clove tips. Drizzle with $\frac{1}{4}$ tsp (1 mL) olive oil and microwave on High for 70 seconds, until fork-tender. Or bake in a pie plate or baking dish at 375°F (190°C) for 15 to 20 minutes, or until fork-tender. *To peel:* Use the flat side of a sharp knife to flatten the clove of garlic. Skin can then be easily removed.

Glaze. To apply a thin, shiny coating to the outside of a baked, sweet or savory food to enhance the appearance and flavor.

Grease pan. See Baking pan.

Griddle. *To test for correct temperature:* Sprinkle a few drops of water on the surface. If the water bounces and dances across the pan, it is ready to use.

Hazelnuts. *To remove skins:* Place hazelnuts in a 350°F (180°C) oven for 15 to 20 minutes. Immediately place in a clean, dry kitchen towel. With your hands, rub the nuts against the towel. Skins will be left in the towel. Be careful: hazelnuts will be very hot.

Hazelnut flour (hazelnut meal). *To make:* See Nut flour.

Herbs. *To store full stems:* Fresh-picked herbs can be stored for up to 1 week with stems standing in water. (Keep leaves out of water.) *To remove leaves:* Remove small leaves from stem by holding the top and running fingers down the stem in the opposite direction of growth. Larger leaves should be snipped off the stem using scissors. *To clean and store fresh leaves:* Rinse under cold running water and spin-dry in a lettuce spinner. If necessary, dry between layers of paper towels. Place a dry paper towel along with the clean herbs in a plastic bag in the refrigerator. Use within 2 to 3 days. Freeze or dry for longer storage. *To measure:* Pack leaves tightly into correct measure. *To snip:* After measuring, transfer to a small glass and cut using the tips of sharp kitchen shears/scissors to avoid bruising the tender leaves. *To dry:* Tie fresh-picked herbs together in small bunches and hang upside down in a well-ventilated location with low humidity and out of sunlight until the leaves are brittle and fully dry. If they turn brown (rather than stay green), the air is too hot. Once fully dried, strip leaves off the stems for storage. Store whole herbs in an airtight container in a cool dark place for up to 1 year and crushed herbs for up to 6 months. (Dried herbs are stored in the dark to prevent the color from fading.) Before using, check herbs and discard any that have faded, lost flavor or smell old and musty. *To dry using a microwave:* Place $\frac{1}{2}$ to 1 cup (125 to 250 mL) herbs between layers of paper towels. Microwave on High for 3 minutes, checking often to be sure they are not scorched. Then microwave for 10-second periods until leaves are brittle and can be pulled from stems easily. *To freeze:* Lay whole herbs in a single layer on a flat surface in the freezer for 2 to 4 hours. Leave whole and pack in plastic bags. Herbs will keep in the freezer for 2 to 3 months. Crumble frozen leaves directly into the dish. Herb leaves are also easier to chop when frozen. Use frozen leaves only for flavoring and not for garnishing, as they lose their crispness when thawed. Some herbs, such as chives, have a very weak flavor when dried, and do not freeze well, but they do grow well inside on a windowsill.

Leeks. *To clean:* Trim roots and wilted green ends. Peel off tough outer layer. Cut leeks in half lengthwise and rinse under cold running water, separating the leaves so the water gets between the layers. Trim individual leaves at the point where they start to become dark in color and course in texture — this will be higher up on the plant the closer you get to the center.

Mix. To combine two or more ingredients uniformly by stirring or using an electric mixer on a low speed.

Nut flour (nut meal). *To make:* Toast nuts (see Nuts), cool to room temperature and grind in a food processor or blender to desired consistency. *To make using ground nuts:* Bake at 350°F (180°C) for 6 to 8 minutes, cool to room temperature and grind finer.

Nuts. *To toast:* Spread nuts in a single layer on a baking sheet and bake at 350°F (180°C) for 6 to 8 minutes, shaking the pan frequently, until fragrant and lightly browned. (Or microwave, uncovered, on High for 1 to 2 minutes, stirring every 30 seconds.) Nuts will darken upon cooling.

Olives. *To pit:* Place olives under the flat side of a large knife; push down on knife until pit pops out.

Onions. *To caramelize:* In a nonstick frying pan, heat 1 tbsp (15 mL) oil over medium heat. Add 2 cups (500 mL) sliced or chopped onions; cook slowly until soft and caramel-colored. If necessary, add 1 tbsp (15 mL) water or white wine to prevent sticking while cooking.

Peaches. *To blanch:* See Blanch.

Pecan flour (pecan meal). *To make:* See Nut flour.

Pine nuts. *To toast:* see Nuts.

Pumpkin seeds. *To toast:* See Sunflower seeds.

Quinoa. *To cook:* For 1 cup (250 mL) cooked quinoa, bring to a boil $\frac{1}{4}$ cup (50 mL) quinoa and $\frac{3}{4}$ cup (175 mL) water. Reduce heat to low; cover and simmer for 18 to 20 minutes, or until water is absorbed and quinoa is tender. Quinoa is cooked when grains turn from white to transparent and the tiny spiral-like germ is separated.

Raisins. *To plump:* Measure a spirit (usually brandy) into a liquid measuring cup and add raisins; microwave on High for 1 minute and let cool.

Sauté. To cook quickly in a small amount of fat at high temperature.

Sesame seeds. *To toast:* See Sunflower seeds.

Sunflower seeds. *To toast:* Spread seeds in a single layer on a baking sheet and bake at 350°F (180°C) for 6 to 10 minutes, shaking the pan frequently, until lightly browned. (Or microwave, uncovered, on High for 1 to 2 minutes, stirring every 30 seconds.) Seeds will darken upon cooling.

Water bath. Place filled jars, with finger-tightened lids, upright on a rack in a boiling water bath canner filled with enough boiling water so that jars are covered by at least 1 inch (2.5 cm) hot water. Cover canner and return to a full, rolling boil. Boil for time specified in recipe.

Whip. To beat ingredients vigorously to increase volume and incorporate air, typically using a whisk or electric mixer. See also Egg whites.

Whipping (35%) cream. *For greater volume:* Chill beaters and bowl in refrigerator for at least 1 hour before whipping.

Wild rice. *To cook:* Rinse 1 cup (250 mL) wild rice under cold running water. Add along with 6 cups (1.5 L) water to a large saucepan. Bring to a boil and cook, uncovered, at a gentle boil for about 35 minutes. Reduce heat, cover and cook for 10 minutes, or until rice is soft but not mushy. Makes 3 cups (750 mL). Store in refrigerator for up to 1 week.

Zest. *To zest:* Use a zester, the fine side of a box grater or a small sharp knife to peel off thin strips of the colored part of the skin of citrus fruits. Be sure not to remove the bitter white pith below.

Celiac Groups

CANADA

Canadian Celiac Association
National Office
5170 Dixie Road, Suite 204
Mississauga, Ontario L4W 1E3
Phone: 800-363-7296
Fax: 905-507-4673
Website: www.celiac.ca

UNITED STATES

Celiac Disease Foundation
13251 Ventura Boulevard, # 1
Studio City, California 91604
Phone: 818-990-2354
Fax: 818-990-2379
Website: www.celiac.org

CSA/USA, Inc.
Celiac Sprue Association
P.O. Box 31700
Omaha, Nebraska 68131-0700
Phone: 877-CSA-4CSA
Fax: 402-558-1347
Website: www.csaceliacs.org

The Gluten Intolerance Group
  of North America (GIG)
15110-10th Avenue SW, Suite A
Seattle, Washington 98166
Phone: 206-246-6652
Fax: 206-246-6531
Website: www.gluten.net

Library and Archives Canada Cataloguing in Publication

Washburn, Donna
The best gluten-free family cookbook / Donna Washburn & Heather Butt.

Includes index.
ISBN 0-7788-0111-X

1. Gluten-free diet–Recipes. I. Butt, Heather II. Title.

RM237.86.W37 2005   641.5'638   C2004-906541-6

Index